RUNNER'S WORLD

RUN TO LOSE

Also by Jennifer Van Allen & Pamela Nisevich Bede:

*The Runner's World Big Book of Marathon
and Half-Marathon Training*

The Runner's World Big Book of Running for Beginners

RUNNER'S WORLD®

RUN TO LOSE

A Complete Guide to
WEIGHT LOSS
for Runners

Jennifer Van Allen and
Pamela Nisevich Bede, RD, CSSD

RODALE.

RODALE *wellness*

Live happy. Be healthy. Get inspired.

Sign up today to get exclusive access to our authors, exclusive bonuses,
and the most authoritative, useful, and cutting-edge information on health,
wellness, fitness, and living your life to the fullest.

Visit us online at RodaleWellness.com
Join us at RodaleWellness.com/Join

Copyright © 2015 by Rodale Inc.

All rights reserved. No part of this publication may be reproduced or transmitted in any form or by any means, electronic or mechanical, including photocopying, recording, or any other information storage and retrieval system, without the written permission of the publisher.

Rodale books may be purchased for business or promotional use or for special sales. For information, please write to:
Special Markets Department, Rodale Inc., 733 Third Avenue,
New York, NY 10017

Printed in the United States of America
Rodale Inc. makes every effort to use acid-free ♾, recycled paper ♻.

Exercise photos: Beth Bischoff
Author photos (page 296): Peter Van Allen for Jennifer Van Allen's photo
and John Segesta for Pamela Nisevich Bede's photo

Book design by Carol Angstadt

Library of Congress Cataloging-in-Publication Data is on file with the publisher.

ISBN 978–1–62336–599–8   paperback

Distributed to the trade by Macmillan

6   8   10   9   7   paperback

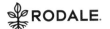

Follow us @RodaleBooks on 🐦 📘 📌 📷

We inspire and enable people to improve their lives and the world around them.
rodalewellness.com

To Jason, Miller, Hunter, Noah, and Peter.
For all your love and support.

CONTENTS

PART I: What to Eat

PART II: How Much to Eat

PART III: When to Eat

INTRODUCTION

It is often said that weight loss is a simple matter of consuming fewer calories than your body burns.

If that sentence made you want to throw this book out the window, you are not alone. Anyone who has tried to lose weight by consuming fewer calories than they burn knows that it's by no means that simple. And it certainly isn't easy. Sure, for a lucky few, the unwanted pounds just melt off as soon as they start exercising more and cutting back on calories. But for many more of us—and close to 6 in 10 Americans want to lose weight, according to a Gallup poll[1]—the process of reaching a feel-great weight is much more confusing. And frustrating.

If only it *were* as simple as calories in, calories out. If it were, we probably wouldn't have an obesity crisis. And those Gallup numbers would look much different.

One could get whiplash trying to keep up with the barrage of diet trends. It seems like every day, someone is making a bold new claim about some sort of superfood—green tea, chia seeds, coconut oil, lemon juice, hot peppers—and the weight-loss magic it performs. Just as dizzying is the list of ingredients we're told to avoid—gluten, meat, wheat, carbs, fats, sugar, fruit, seeds, or acidic foods. It's hard to keep up—much less figure out how to make the scale move.

And if you're running to lose weight, or trying to lose weight while training for a race, it's even more difficult to wade through the tidal waves of advice to figure out how to shrink your waistline and your race times. So often, nutrition guidance for runners contradicts even the most conventional dieting advice.

What's all this about fueling up for a run?

Why on earth would you go out and eat more calories to prepare for a workout designed to burn off the calories you already consumed?

And if weight loss is just a matter of consuming fewer calories and incinerating more, the idea of consuming calories *during* a run, where you're trying to burn them, sounds downright ludicrous.

And what about carbs?

Dieters everywhere are cutting them to shed weight.

But runners are told to make carbs more than half their daily calories.

And running and training for a race introduces so many other questions and variables.

Does a 3-mile run mean you get to eat 300 extra calories that day?

If you run 6 miles, do you deserve a brownie?

No wonder there's so much confusion.

There certainly was for Steve Lambert, a 33-year-old father of two who lost more than 100 pounds with the help of Weight Watchers and a half-marathon training program.

"When I was training, my Weight Watchers mind was telling me not to use anything during training runs or the race, but my body was telling me I needed fuel after 1.5 hours of running," says Lambert, a planner from Virginia Beach. Ultimately he took the advice of running buddies and went for an energy bar during long runs. "It worked perfectly," he says, "but subconsciously I was worrying about how many points I was consuming that day."

For others, like Rob Walter, a 40-year-old father of two, the confusion leads to a frustrating process of training harder and harder, restricting more and more, only to see the scale—and race times—come to a standstill.

Walter was looking to get faster, feel more comfortable in his jeans, and shave about 20 pounds from his 6'1" frame. So he tried various high-protein and low-carb approaches while training for half-marathons and marathons. But nothing lasted more than a few weeks. "I would feel like total crap before, during, and after workouts," says Walter, a CFO from Dublin, Ohio. "I had zero energy, and my cravings were horrendous because the bread and carbs I loved were discouraged."

Others, like Lynn Ramsey, a 45-year-old mother of two from Seattle, find that no matter how many miles they run, the scale only moves in the wrong direction.

The more Ramsey ran, the hungrier she became. She once gained 10 pounds training for a marathon. While training for, then recovering from, the Marine Corps Marathon, she remembers being hungry basically from September 2011 to February 2012.

"I hate dieting, counting calories, depriving myself," says Ramsey. "And I get really hungry as my mileage increases."

She's not alone. In one study of 64 marathon trainees, some runners lost as much as 27 pounds; others gained as much as 14 pounds. And these people weren't slow; the average finish time was 4:25. Some 63 percent of the subjects said they ate more during training.[2]

We've heard from thousands of these runners at *Runner's World*. So many runners are confused.

For all of them, the pain and frustration of having extra pounds to shed are more difficult than any physical discomforts involved in making their legs and lungs stronger.

After several failed attempts at weight loss, Lambert says, "I just sort of brainwashed and said, 'Hey, I am an athletic fat guy; that is what I am.' I pretended that being overweight was okay. I pretended that I could just go to the gym a few times a week, and barely doing anything would make a difference."

A few years ago, it became clear that it wouldn't: "My sleep wasn't efficient, I was out of breath tying my shoes, and just everyday stuff was hard," he says. "I realized that I needed to be healthy so I could enjoy life."

Yes, the lighter you are, the more efficiently you'll run, the more enjoyable running will feel, and the faster you'll finish. Weight can affect performance in running more than in other sports, such as cycling and swimming.[3]

Wesley Cure, a 31-year-old runner who lost 75 pounds to reach his high school weight, learned this firsthand.

"When I first started running, it really hurt my shins," he says. "After I lost 15 or 20 pounds, that pain stopped. After that, my speed increase seemed to be in direct correlation to my weight loss. I generally just felt healthier; I had more energy and I *was* faster."

But losing weight and getting faster don't always happen in this tidy upward progression—not even for those like Cure, who ran a 3:10 in his first marathon. He struggled to find where and how treats could fit into his regular diet. After months of swearing off sweets, "I ended up bingeing once and realized there was no way I could go without these things," he says. "To try to give up the occasional sweets and greasy meal just wasn't realistic for me. So I eat a little so I don't want a lot."

Indeed, this struggle isn't just an issue for those who are clinically overweight. Runners from all parts of the pack struggle to juggle their racing and weight-loss goals. Shedding weight while also getting the fuel you need to log a peak performance just isn't easy.

It certainly wasn't easy for Olympian and 2015 USA Marathon champ Blake Russell, who became one of the nation's leading marathoners while becoming a mother. Resuming her professional running life meant losing the 40 pounds she gained with each of her children. While there are many tales of elites who run all the way to labor and delivery, Russell took months off her training with each pregnancy.

"I did not run much because, well, the weight came on fast, and it's not fun to run when you are miserable," she says. When she tried to run during her second pregnancy, with her 3-year-old son in the baby jogger, "he would ask me why we were going so slow, or why I was walking?"

Eating for recovery—focusing on carbs, protein, and fat to help her recover, as well as hydration—helped her regain her fitness and speed without getting hurt. But so did a few key phrases: a note on the scale at her doctor's office that read "This scale measures weight, not worth; you are worthy and beautiful." Plus sage words from her coach.

"He always said that talent doesn't go away," she says. "These words echoed in my head, and frankly, I clung to them as I was whipping myself into shape. Some days the workouts were terrible because I was exhausted. Other days I saw a glimmer of my old self. Most days it was nice to get outside and have some *me* time, a rarity when you are a mother. It helped that I remembered what it felt like to feel fit and fast. I wanted that feeling again."

She got that feeling again, winning the 2015 Los Angeles Marathon and the USA Marathon Championship.

When she stepped up to the starting line, her heart was pounding. "My only thought was 'I just want to see what I can do,'" she says. "It felt more like a race against myself. I knew that runner was in there somewhere, and I just had to find a way to bring her out once again. I am glad I remembered what it was like to feel fit and fast, and that I wanted that feeling bad enough to work for it. I am thrilled that the hard work paid off, and what's even more thrilling is that I had my family there to share in the victory."

In *Run to Lose*, you will learn how to juggle your weight-loss and training goals to see the numbers you want both on the scale and at the finish line.

But first you must identify your personal roadblocks. Each person has a unique set of obstacles—the habits, temptations, lifestyle, or time and resource constraints—that's getting in the way of their goals.

So the solutions will necessarily be unique for each person.

If you want to lose weight and get faster, only you can identify what your unique difficulties are (there's usually more than one). And only you can identify the approach that will be the best fit for your particular body, age, desires, underlying health issues, cravings, lifestyle, temperament, and family at any given time.

In *Run to Lose*, we'll help you identify those obstacles and get past them. For some people, it's a matter of keeping foods out of sight and out of mind at all times. Steve Lambert had to find a way to keep doughnuts in his diet to avert a binge down the road. Some people swear by calorie-counting apps.

For Kate McPhail, losing more than 100 pounds was a matter of making small, incremental changes, such as swapping whole grain for white bread—and finding healthier items that packed in flavor and didn't make her long for her old meals. "I never decided to eat *x* amount of calories; I just started to make smarter food choices," says McPhail, 31, a nurse from Phoenix. "Instead of sleeves of cookies I would make some homemade, healthy versions."

For Kyle Klaver, a 48-year-old engineer from Charlotte, North Carolina, it was a matter of eliminating processed foods.

"If it comes in a box or a bag, I don't eat it," he says.

Because he travels frequently for work, his plan of attack to reach his weight-loss goals involved scouting out restaurants with healthy options ahead of time on an app and becoming comfortable deconstructing a menu item to eat only what he wants.

"Sometimes the restaurant will allow me to order a dish the way I want, or I just order the standard and tear it apart at the table," he says.

For Rob Walter, it wasn't until he started incorporating the carbs back into his diet that he made a breakthrough on the bathroom scale and at the finish line.

For runner Nikki Marshall, 38, of Melbourne, Australia, the problem wasn't how much she was eating, or when she was eating; food made for a convenient, easy, legal way to blunt the feelings of exhaustion, depletion, and anxiety from having a newborn.

"I was trying to eat my feelings away!" she says.

In *Run to Lose*, you'll learn how to identify the unique obstacles that are keeping *you* from reaching *your* unique weight-loss and running goals. And you'll find all the tools you need to overcome those obstacles.

Start by taking the Run to Lose quiz on page 17 and use the responses to help you navigate the book. Don't worry. There are no right answers— only honest ones. We're not keeping score. Retake the quiz periodically for a gut check. Confused about whether carbs are good or evil? Turn to Chapter 1. Don't know how much to eat? In Part II, you'll find help. Want to rev up your calorie burn but need to keep your workout time short? Find out how in Chapter 24. Do you feel powerless in the face of the box of doughnuts in the office break room? Turn to Chapter 28. And what about stress eating—when the going gets tough, do the tough go for a candy bar? (Chapter 28 can help you with that.) Can green tea boost your calorie burn, even when you're sitting at your desk? (Find out in Chapter 15.) And if you're trying to choose one of the more popular conventional diet plans, or you're already on one, we can help you determine how to integrate that diet into your life (turn to Chapter 14). You can apply the information you learn in this book to any conventional diet or training approach.

Throughout the book, you'll read inspiring stories of runners just like you who struggled then succeeded in finding the Run to Lose diet and training plan that worked for them. Some struggled with sweets. Others needed an education in caloric counts. Portions were a problem for others. Many runners struggled to break the habit of turning to food when they longed for relief from emotional discomforts such as stress, fear, anxiety, and depression. All of them struggled to sort out how to mix and match dieting and training advice to meet their weight-loss and racing goals.

Indeed, running to lose isn't one-size-fits-all—this book is geared to help you design your own diet and running program in a way that works best for you.

That said, there are a few ground rules to follow (see page 9 for those). Your eating and your exercise efforts have to improve the quality of your life and not degrade it. If you can't imagine keeping up these training and eating routines forever, they're not the right ones for you. Ultimately they won't last, and the weight will return.

Rest assured, the time you take to identify your obstacles, and design your own Run to Lose diet and training plan, will be well worth the investment. The rewards go beyond anything that could be measured on the scale or the finish-line clock. Just ask anyone who has done it themselves.

For Kyle Klaver, losing the weight has boosted his confidence. He doesn't hide in the background of pictures. He doesn't get the constant colds he used to. And at the age of 48, he has more energy than ever.

"My energy level is unbelievable," he says. "I used to take naps on

Saturdays and Sundays. Now, even after my long-run days, I feel I could go do it again later in the day. And my mind and memory are better too."

Or take it from Sarah Williarty, a college professor and mother of two from Middletown, Connecticut. She started running to improve her health, but in the process of cutting an hour from her marathon time, breaking 2 hours in the half-marathon, and finally getting rid of that last 5 pounds, she benefited in ways that could never be measured by numbers.

"Getting that much faster made me feel like a rock star and kind of like an athlete," she says. As a self-described bookworm, "those were very new feelings."

What's more, "On other parts of life, I quit being afraid," she says. "I quit being afraid of getting hurt if I tried to run fast. I quit being afraid of talking to other moms. I even started speaking up a lot more at work in professional situations. I started organizing more social events for my family. I kind of feel like I started living in a way that I hadn't before. I had been pulling my punches without realizing it. I don't completely understand what I was worrying about before, and I don't completely understand why I want to run fast now, but I know that the drive to run faster has spilled over into other parts of my life in ways that are very positive. It's given me a lot more confidence."

As you begin your Run to Lose journey, we hope that you gain the benefits that are just as enduring.

YOUR RUN TO LOSE GROUND RULES
Or, the best advice we've ever gotten, or given

We believe that weight loss and running better aren't one-size-fits-all propositions; each person has unique obstacles, and *Run to Lose* is designed to help you learn how to balance your weight-loss and training goals and design your own strategies that best fit your unique needs, lifestyle, temperament, and temptations. At the end of each chapter of *Run to Lose* you will find concrete steps you can take to overcome your personal obstacles.

That said, certain ground rules have been proven to work for anyone. These strategies can help you reach your goals no matter what diet you're on or what your kryptonite food is. Why? Because these behaviors organically foster and nourish the habits that pave the way for weight-loss and running success. Think of them as a healthy version of gateway drugs. They're based on the most enduring lessons we've used and applied from experts who spend their lives researching this stuff. And they're based on the strategies we've found to be most powerful in our work with thousands of runners and dieters over the past 6 years. In the *Runner's World* Challenge, the magazine's online marathon and half-marathon program, and The Starting Line, *Runner's World's* Beginner's Training Program. Rip these pages from our book or mix, match, and make up your own. (See rule #14!)

1. You are an experiment of one. Longtime *Runner's World* columnist and all-around guru George Sheehan said that, and it's true. What works for others may not work for you. No one else has to live your precise life, with your specific challenges, biochemistry, anatomy, injury history, boss, commute, calendar, or minefield of family commitments. Reach for guidance from experts (including us), but the organizing principle of any diet should be how well it works for your unique life. And it should, in some way, fit into your own personal definition of fun and enjoyment. As Anna Quindlen once wrote, "If your success is not on your own terms, if it looks good to the world but does not feel good in your heart, it is not success at all."

2. When something works, excuse-proof it. Running and weight watching are tough enough; make the habits that work for you as easy as possible to practice. Any crazy-making strategy that requires you to twist your life, your family, and other priorities into a pretzel won't last and won't work. So keep tempting foods out of the house, out of sight, and out of mind. If you love running at sunrise but worry about waking the kids on your way out, keep your running gear by the front door or in your car. Need coffee before you go? Invest in the coffeemaker that automatically brews in the morning. Invest in high-quality jackets, shoes, gloves, hats, and fuel belts that allow you to get outside in snow, sleet, rain, and any weather. Believe us, we know, you'll get a little extra runner's high from venturing out in conditions that other people won't even drive in.

3. When something stops working, stop working it. Give any new strategy at least a week before you call it quits. But remember Albert Einstein famously said—that the definition of insanity is doing the same thing over and over again and expecting different results. Sure, it can be scary to diverge from the known, especially when something has worked for you in the past. But if the thought of running the same 3-mile loop is boring you and making it more difficult to get out the door, take a different route. If you're not seeing results from the strength-training routine you've been doing for 2 months, try something else. Likewise, if the same old dinner that helped you shed the first 5 pounds now makes you feel bored, deprived, or constipated or has just stopped tasting good, try something new that matches the nutrient file. (The Internet is awash in healthy recipes designed by people who share your goals—and your dietary restrictions.)

4. Take good notes. When the run goes well, write it down. When the run goes the opposite of well, write it down. Same goes with weight watching. A day of perfect eating? Write it down. A day of careening completely off the rails? Taking notes can be tough, and it can be humiliating to record something you feel shame about. But doing so will ultimately help you. Why? You'll draw confidence from seeing all you accomplished add up, and when the going gets tough, taking a look at those accomplishments will help you restore faith in yourself and remind you that one day is not destiny. Having a record of the good and the bad will also provide important clues you can use to find the culprit when you're getting hurt, gaining weight, or just feeling low. What's more, studies have shown that good notes lead to weight loss. A 2008 study in the *American Journal of Preventive Medicine* found that among 1,700 overweight runners, those who kept a food diary more than 5 days a week lost almost twice as much as those who didn't, and they kept the weight off.[1]

5. Take a time-out. Scientists have shown it can take less than 2 minutes for an urge, a thought, or a craving to disappear from your consciousness. Many mindful eating experts, like Dr. Susan Albers, a Cleveland Clinic psychologist and author of seven books, including the *New York Times* bestselling *Eat.Q.: Unlock the Weight-Loss Power of Emotional Intelligence*, have recommended that dieters use this to their advantage. (Read more about mindful eating in Chapter 30.) If you're hammering away at a frustrating work assignment and thinking "potato chips," rather than engaging in a wrestling match with your willpower, or automatically inserting hand into bag, tell yourself you can have the chips, in 2 minutes. Set a timer to chime in 2 minutes, then do something else. (Brushing your teeth, walking around the block, or refilling a water bottle are good options.) Chances are, by the time you hear the timer chime the chips won't seem so compelling anymore. Other research has confirmed that distraction works. A study performed by mindless eating expert Dr. Brian Wansink found that when people were given just a few bites of a snack they wanted, then distracted for 15 minutes, they were just as satisfied as other people who had been given bigger portions.[2]

6. Follow the celery rule. It's often difficult to separate a mental craving from true physical hunger. When you're truly ravenous, even a celery stick will do. When you're craving something, it's typically very specific—like the rush of a piece of chocolate or the salty crunch of a potato chip—and you're probably hankering for relief from something deeper—boredom, frustration, loneliness, fear, a work deadline, a quandary with a loved one, etc. No matter what you do or how much you eat, that feeling is still going to be there when you finish eating. It will only be compounded by feelings of remorse about what you just ate.

7. Get outside. Research has proven it: Time spent in nature relieves stress, boosts mood, and combats depression. In a study published in the June 2014 issue of *Journal of Environmental Psychology*,[3] participants who spent time in a wooded, natural setting felt more restored and had better moods, more creativity and vitality, and lower levels of cortisol (the stress hormone) compared to those who spent time in an urban setting. Even if you're not running—and especially on days when you're not scheduled to exercise—it's important to get at least 10 minutes of outside time, sipping in fresh air, hearing the tweeting birds, and looking at trees, grass, and flowers. If you set the bar low—say 10 minutes—chances are, by the time the 10-minute chime goes off, you'll want to keep going.

8. Reach out. Have a circle of people who can and will genuinely help you celebrate your successes and commiserate when things don't go so well. They can be online or on the ground. Research has shown that social connection helps seal success. A study published in the May 2012 issue of *Obesity* found that in a program where 34 percent of participants lost at least 5 percent of their body weight, a powerful factor was "social influence"; that is, the fact that close friends with similar goals acted as a team, worked out together, and exchanged pep-talk e-mails.[4] However low or lost you feel, you can be assured that someone out there has felt the same way at some point. (And see rule #10.)

9. Act like the person you want to be. Ghandi said "Be the change you want to see in the world," and when it comes to weight loss and running, it really does work. Think of the person you'd like to be or someone you admire—who has succeeded in weight loss or reached a PR. And when you start waffling over whether you should get the heck outside or stick your hand in a bag of pretzels for stress relief, consider what the person you aspire to be, or the person you most admire, would do. (For more on this, see Chapter 30.)

10. When you get lost, ask for directions. Connect with others, online or on the ground. There is so much free help out there. Contact us directly at RuntoLose.com. We will answer your e-mails. Researchers have spent hundreds of years studying what works and what doesn't, and people (like us) spend our lives helping other people with obstacles like yours reach goals like yours. We are so lucky to live in an age where we can connect with others and with experts in just a few keystrokes. Take advantage of that.

11. Compromise, don't sacrifice. Any healthy way of eating or exercising will expand your life, not contract it. Yes, long runs will inevitably nibble away at your family and work time. But on a whole, sustainable eating and exercise habits should help you meet new people, explore places you've never seen, open your perspective, or live longer so you can enjoy more quality time with your loved ones. When your eating and exercise habits are contracting your life—making you feel deprived, lonely, isolated, and like you're being forced to make uncomfortable sacrifices—those strategies will not work, and they will not last. This is particularly important with your eating habits. Your eating habits should pave the way for you to try new fruits, veggies, grains, recipes, and ways of cooking you've never tried before. If you feel limited, deprived, and confined, and your daily meals feel like punishment, it's important to change something.

12. Be nice. That goes for yourself and others. Trying to beat your body, your will, or someone else into submission just doesn't work. Studies have shown that people who are compassionate with others feel better and avert binges, while those with negative self-talk do not. A study published in the 2007 issue of the *Journal of Social and Clinical Psychology* found that after indulging in a doughnut, dieters with self-compassion could monitor and hold back further eating, more so than those who focused on the negative implications of the indulgence.[5] If, after an off-the-diet cookie, your mind and heart swell with feelings of hopelessness, self-hatred, and regret, chances are, you'll resign yourself to failure, throw your hands up, and in an effort to feel better, eat the whole bag. (See Chapter 28 for more on this.) But if you imagine you're counseling a friend who just ate the same cookie, you would be more likely to assure that friend that one cookie won't ruin a diet and that everyone goes off track sometimes. If you look at your food or training log, you'll see that 99 percent of the time you're doing great; you can start again and get back on track right away. You can calm down and put the cookies away. The same goes for running. This is why rule #4 is so important. If you hit the wall before finishing one day's run and have to shuffle home, the demoralization can be paralyzing, and it can take days to get the courage to hit the road again. But if you look at your log and see how many miles you've covered, or days you've run, you'll see that one bad day is no big deal in light of all you've accomplished.

13. Set up nonfood rewards. Make a list of five things you can buy or do to celebrate your success. These all should be completely unrelated to food, as rewarding yourself with a muffin the size of a volleyball is never a good idea. (See Chapter 30 on mindless eating.) Likewise, you don't want to wait until you accomplish some mileage milestone to get new shoes. Buy a book. Buy a new shirt. Get a manicure. Get a massage. Make a date to see friends. Plan a trip. It can be anything.

14. Make your own rules. (See rule #1.) Take these rules to heart, but set up rules that personally suit your goals and needs and help you overcome your unique obstacles. You may have a rule of "no computers in the kitchen" so you don't get in the habit of "eating and working." You may have a rule of making your home a chocolate-free zone to avoid temptation, or no-eating-in-the-car rules. Have a "recess rule" that requires you to go outside every day for emotional and mental benefits. (See rule #7.) After you take the Run to Lose quiz, read this book, and take the quiz again, make up your own ground rules that set you up for success. Think of them as the most valuable pieces of advice you'd give a loved one who was sharing your struggle.

RUN TO LOSE SELF-QUIZ

You may have a sense of what's keeping you from reaching your weight-loss goals or you may just feel mystified, frustrated, and downright stuck. In *Run to Lose*, we'll help you identify your weaknesses and figure out how to get stronger. Start by taking this quiz; read it before you dive into the book.

Don't worry; no one is keeping score. There's no right answer. There are only honest answers. The Run to Lose quiz is meant to help you reflect on where you're getting stalled, so you can more efficiently and effectively find the tools you need to break through. Let the answers to this quiz guide you to the chapters in the book that are most relevant to you. And to determine where there's room for improvement, return to it anytime you hit roadblocks or plateaus.

1. Age:

2. Current weight:

3. Goal weight:

4. Body fat percentage (if known):

5. Goal body fat percentage (if applicable):

6. Goal race time and distance:

7. Current race time and distance:

8. Do you have any chronic medical conditions?

9. Do you take any prescribed medications that may impact your weight?

10. Do you have any limitations to your physical activity?

11. Do you have any medical conditions or allergies that impact what you eat?

12. Do you take any vitamins or supplements? If so, which ones and why?

13. What is your motivation for wanting to lose weight?

14. Worst eating habit:

15. Healthiest eating habit:

16. How many alcoholic drinks do you consume per week?

17. How many nights per week do you eat out?

18. How many nights per week do you cook at home?

19. How frequently do you eat fruits and vegetables?

20. How frequently do you skip meals?

21. How frequently do you eat breakfast?

22. Do you track your calories or your intake of carbs, fats, and protein?

23. Do you read food labels on packaged goods?

24. Do you keep a food journal?

25. Do you weigh yourself regularly? If so, how frequently?

26. Do you measure your weight loss in some other way—say, a favorite pair of pants?

27. How many times a week do you work out?

28. Do you regularly do faster-paced runs like tempo work and speedwork?

29. Do you strength train? If so, how often?

30. Do you cross-train?

31. Do you measure how fast, how far, and how long you run?

32. What's your favorite type of workout?

33. What's your least favorite workout?

34. Do you keep a training journal?

35. If so, which metrics do you track?

36. Have you been sidelined for more than 2 weeks by running-related injuries?

37. Did you eat less, the same, or more during the time you were sidelined?

38. How often do you get outside for exercise or otherwise?

39. How many hours per day do you sit? (in a car, at your office, etc.)

40. Do you enjoy any physical activities other than running and do them on a regular basis?

41. What diets have you tried?

42. Which elements of those diets have worked?

43. Which elements of those diets have not worked?

44. Have you, or are you currently, eliminating any entire food groups—not related to a medical condition, but purely for the sake of weight loss?

45. Do you ever eat when you're not hungry—because you're bored, sad, happy, angry, lonely, procrastinating, restless, or enduring some other uncomfortable emotion?

46. Do you ever eat food just because it's there?

47. If you could surgically remove one bad eating habit from yourself, what would it be?

48. Do you do any contemplative, self-reflection exercises on a regular basis, like writing or meditation?

49. Do you have anyone with whom you can connect about your weight-loss struggles, either online or in person?

50. Do you have a fitness or running role model? What kinds of eating and exercise habits do they practice?

MEASURING SUCCESS
You've likely seen advice to throw out your scale

And yes, the scale should not be the only tool you use to measure success. A variety of factors that have nothing to do with your speed or eating habits can drive the scale skyward, throw off your race times, and drive you absolutely nuts. We live and die by these numbers, and they can make us swell with confidence we never thought possible, or send us reeling into dark caves of depression. After all, who wants to spend precious hours and days trying to eat right and run better, if, according to the numbers, it's not working? That depression can be pretty powerful, driving us to resign ourselves to a "why bother?" state of mind, blow off our next workout, or drown our sorrows in a family-size bag of chocolate chips.

When it comes to numbers, here's what we think: Tracking progress works. But single tools, when used in isolation—whether it's the scale, the finish-line clock, your training watch, a body-composition test, blood pressure and cholesterol levels, or even the number next to the

CHEW ON THIS

Even the highest-tech gadget can't detect the most important measures of success—such as your confidence, your efficacy at work, and the happiness of your loved ones. Regardless of what any electronic readout says, the miles you run and the food you eat should improve your quality of life, not degrade it. If your family is feeling neglected, your boss is ticked off, or you just feel upset or deprived all the time, none of those metrics matters. So as you're looking at the numbers, try not to lose sight of the big picture: Your own happiness, the contentment of your loved ones, and the causes and work you care about count for a lot.

word "size" on your favorite pants—can't completely reveal important parts of the story: how much fitness you're gaining and how you feel.

Because each metric has its limitations, and because progress rarely occurs as a straightforward, upward trajectory, it's wise to measure as many metrics as possible without risking obsession and compulsion. That way, your sense of satisfaction and accomplishment from all the hard work you do isn't completely dependent on a single measure, which could be way off for any variety of factors that have nothing to do with what you're consuming, or what you're doing on the road. Using three to five metrics, which you can take at a variety of different frequencies, is a good place to start.

Here are some key measures of success, and how to work with them.

Your Mileage and Pace

Why it matters: It's important to ramp up mileage and speed very gradually to prevent injury and allow the body to adapt to new stresses and get stronger. In general you don't want to increase either metric by more than 10 percent from one week to another. Taking good notes on how many miles you ran, your pace, how you felt, and the shoes you wore can help you detect injuries or signs of burnout before they derail you.

How often: Every day.

What it leaves out: What you're eating. If you're eating back all the calories you burned (aka overcompensating) after every workout, you're likely undoing any potential weight-loss benefits you're getting from your workouts. By the same token, if you're restricting your calories or carbs too much, going into every run feeling depleted, and hitting the wall before you finish the day's mileage, you're handicapping your workouts before you even hit the road. While a training journal has some clues about what's helping—or hurting—your weight-loss efforts, what you're eating is a huge part of it.

The Scale

Why it matters: Trying to change something specific without tracking whether that specific something is changing is an invitation for frustration and delusion. In one of the key findings of the National Weight Control Registry, a long-term study of those who have lost an average of 66 pounds and kept it off for at least 5 years, 75 percent of participants weighed themselves at least once a week.[1] Many of the headlines that urge you to throw out the scale are warnings about its limitations. And those should be real considerations. Your body weight can fluctuate throughout the day and between days due to factors that have nothing to do with what you're eating or how fast you're running. Those factors can include hormones, dehydration, the amount of carbs or sodium in your last meal, or even constipation.

When: First thing in the morning, naked, after you go to the bathroom but before you eat or drink anything.

How often: No more than once a day. Given how many factors can make your weight fluctuate, weighing yourself any more often is a waste of time. (The exception is if you're using this to take the "sweat test" [see Chapter 8 on what to drink] to figure out how much fluid you need for your workout.)

What it leaves out: Whether you're getting faster and how much you're improving your body composition by increasing your muscle mass and decreasing your body fat percentage. The scale also doesn't measure whether your blood pressure, cholesterol, and risk of chronic disease are all heading in the right direction.

Body Composition (Body Fat Percentage)

Why it matters: Reducing your body fat and improving lean muscle mass can help you run faster, burn more calories even when you're not running, and improve your overall health. By the same token, not enough fat can lead to injury and other health complications. For men, ideal body fat is 8 to 24 percent; for women, the ideal is 21 to 35 percent. For some athletes, it's going to be even lower. The most accurate measurements are DEXA scan or Bod Pod scan, which are offered at some hospitals, research centers, doctors' offices, gyms, and universities. They do cost money. Other methods are easier and more accessible, but they're less accurate. Special scales offered at some gyms offer a body fat measurement based on bioelectrical impedance analysis.

When: At the start of your workout or weight-loss efforts. At a gym, a personal trainer can use calipers to measure skinfold thickness in the chest, belly, triceps, and thighs. These can be accurate if the trainer using the calipers has experience, uses high-quality equipment, and uses the right equation to translate those measurements into an estimate of body fat.

How often: As your training progresses and as you make improvements, checking in on your body comp can be a great pat on the back. You might consider getting your body comp checked as you move from one cycle of training to another, say at the beginning of your marathon training program, then just before the race.

What it leaves out: How you feel, any dietary changes, and how fast you're running. It also doesn't give you a sense of your risk of chronic diseases.

How Fast You're Running

Why it matters: The same thing we said about the scale applies here: If your goal is to get faster, it's important to track your pace to get a sense of how fast you're going.

When: On any run.

How often: On every run.

What it leaves out: If the weather is hot, humid, you're injured, or you didn't get any sleep the night before, your pace is likely to slow, and your level of effort is sure to spike. It also doesn't directly measure how you feel on each run (though if you feel awful on a run, your average pace probably will reflect that; see Chapter 27 on measuring your running efforts). Your running pace also doesn't measure any dietary changes that could be improving or derailing your running efforts or lowering or raising your risk of chronic disease.

5-K Times

Why it matters: In a 5-K race setting, you're running at the fastest pace you can sustain. This is a great way to measure your aerobic fitness and running performance. It's also a great way to practice and test out your racing and fueling tactics. And because the race itself involves a very small time commitment, and the training required can be as little as 20 miles a week, it's a very accessible way to measure your fitness. What's more, because races typically offer aid stations, cheering spectators, a measured course, and automated timing, you're set up for success. Try to find races on courses with similar elevation profiles to use throughout the season. Some running clubs have race series on the same course so you can fairly measure your fitness gains. That's ideal, because if one 5-K race is on a flat course and your next race is on a hilly course, you won't be able to fairly compare your times.

When: At the beginning of your fitness program.

How often: Every 6 to 8 weeks.

What it leaves out: If your diet is still out of whack, it's not going to show up immediately in your 5-K results. Because factors such as wind, heat, and the elevation profile of the race course can all impact your race times, the time at the finish-line clock will not always be a direct reflection of your fitness or the dietary changes you're making.

Resting Heart Rate

Why it matters: If your heart isn't healthy, it's likely that your running, weight-loss, and overall health goals are going to remain out of reach. As you get fitter and build your aerobic power, your heart is not going to have to work as hard as it did before. Think about climbing the stairs. When you're unfit, at the top of the stairs you're likely to feel out of breath, with your heart pounding hard and fast in a panicky twitter. As you strengthen your heart through running, with each beat your heart can pump more blood. The heart doesn't have to beat as many times as it did before to get you the blood you need to power your body up the stairs. So as you get fitter, your resting heart rate should go down.

When: First thing in the morning. Before you get out of bed. Take your pulse for 1 minute and write it down.

How often: Daily.

What it leaves out: If the weather is hot, you're stressed, sick, sleep-deprived, or in any other condition, your resting heart rate may be affected. It also doesn't measure your dietary improvements or any changes in your body composition.

Your Pants

Why it matters: Your pants can offer a good assessment of whether you're trimming your waistline and whittling away the belly fat that is linked to so many chronic diseases. They can also offer a big confidence boost, which counts for a lot. There is no better feeling than knowing you can fit into your "skinny" jeans. And nothing can keep you more honest than how you feel in your pants.

When: Before you have eaten; ideally first thing in the morning.

How often: Once a week.

What it leaves out: Whether you're getting faster, how much you weigh, or your overall health.

Your Carbs, Fats, Protein (Macronutrients)

Why it matters: Runners need all three macronutrients to run well. Diets that eliminate one group of nutrients altogether just can't give you the fuel you need to run your best, unleash your fitness potential, and ultimately lose weight. For instance, if you try to completely cut out fats, which help the body absorb vitamins and minerals among other important physiologic functions, you set yourself up for nutrient deficiencies and injury. If you try to completely cut out carbs, you starve your body of its best energy source for running and set yourself up to run out of energy well before you're done with your runs. By counting macronutrients, you can ensure you're getting all the nutrients you need to run well.

When: At every meal.

How often: Every day.

What it leaves out: The quality of the food you're consuming. As noted in Chapter 1, you can meet these targets and still be consuming foods that aren't going to ultimately help your waistline, your race times, or your long-term health. Sure, with 20 grams of protein, that protein bar can help you meet your daily protein target, but it's not going to satisfy you and offer you the nutrition or the sense of satiation that, say, the 20 grams in healthier foods such as egg whites, tuna, or even Greek yogurt does.

Calories

Why it matters: Yes, weight loss is more than just calories in and calories out. But it can help to know how many calories you need to fuel your running and what your daily calorie limits should ideally be in order to lose weight. (Your best bet is to work with a registered dietitian or sports dietitian to determine what your daily calorie target should be. If that's not possible, use the formulas on pages 156 to 157 in

Chapter 16 to get a general idea.) Even just the process of counting calories and looking up how many calories each food contains can be eye-opening. You might find that the fast-food breakfast you weren't thinking much about actually loads you up with a day's worth of calories before you even get to your morning meeting. And you may see that the bag of trail mix you don't even enjoy and could definitely do without is inflating your daily calorie intake unnecessarily. Studies have shown that people drastically underestimate the number of calories any food contains.[2] And the more calories a food contains, the more drastically they tend to underestimate the calories.

When: At first, try tracking your calories for 1 week to get a sense of how many you're consuming at present, and keep a food log. There are lots of free calorie-tracking Web sites and apps on the market. This may be an eye-opener, and it may give you a clue about where your weight-loss obstacles are.

How often: Daily.

What it leaves out: Not all calories are created equal. Counting the number of calories you're taking in does not take into consideration the quality of those calories and the nutrition they provide. Some calories—say those from sugar and processed foods—can rev up your appetite and set you up to hit the wall both in your races and at your afternoon staff meeting. Other calories—say those from whole grains, fruits, and veggies—offer a variety of nutrients and minerals, keep your GI system working efficiently, and keep you feeling full and satisfied until your next meal. The sheer volume of calories you're consuming also doesn't say anything about the quality of your workouts, your body composition, or your risk of chronic diseases.

Your Personal Healthy Habits

Why it matters: Each person has his or her own unique blend of practices that help them feel happy and keep them on track every day. (See Part V on "Why We Eat.") Scientists often call these *process goals*.

They're the steps in the process that help you achieve the results you're seeking. If you watch them accumulate, they keep you honest. If you don't see your weight or paces change, you can take a look at these habits and see where you've been diligent and where you've been lax. By the same token, you can draw confidence from all the healthy habits you're practicing on a regular basis, when the scale and your pace don't seem to be budging. Here are some examples: Keeping a journal each day may help eliminate the stress that drives you to eat. Keeping track of the water you drink might help you stay hydrated and improve how you feel on your runs, and how fast you go. If nighttime eating is a problem, keeping track of the number of times you close the kitchen after dinner might build your confidence.

When: As soon as possible.

How often: As often as possible.

What it leaves out: Your healthy habits may not match up with how you feel about the numbers on the scale or the finish-line clock. But they will pay off in the long run. And if the other numbers aren't reflecting success, you can always draw confidence from seeing how long and how well you've reversed unhealthy habits. If you stick with healthy process goals, eventually your weight and your race times will cooperate.

Lynn's Story: **Measuring Success**

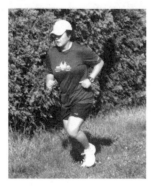

LYNN RAMSEY has been contending with weight issues since she was a toddler. Her intake was monitored so closely, she remembers having to hide what she ate as a young child. When she was a teenager, her parents paid her to go to diet and exercise classes geared for adult women, and they bought her summer gym memberships.

"I really cannot remember when my size and weight were not an issue," she says.

Over time she got into running and

eventually finished about a dozen marathons, 24 half-marathons, and countless other shorter races, losing and regaining weight many times along the way. But running wasn't the magic bullet for weight loss that it is for some people—her weight varied from 175 to 155 as she was training and competing. If anything, the longer distances made weight loss more challenging.

"I hate dieting, counting calories, depriving myself, and I get really hungry as my mileage increases," says Ramsey, 45, a mother of two. While training for, then recovering from, the Marine Corps Marathon, she remembers feeling hungry basically from September 2011 to February 2012.

In recent years, she has been able to sustain her weight within a healthy 5-to-10-pound range with a series of small, sustainable changes.

She taught herself to drink unsweetened iced tea instead of diet soda. She takes her coffee black. When ordering salad at a restaurant, she orders dressing on the side and dips her fork in it. She orders sides of broccoli and sweet potatoes. And she stopped finishing off her kids' meals.

"It's little things like this that I have done over time that just became a part of my normal life," she says. "I am able to enjoy life and not feel deprived or constantly worry about counting calories, points, or if a food is acceptable or not."

But the biggest breakthrough has been in her way of thinking about weight.

"The most important change I made when it comes to weight loss and running is changing my mind-set," she says. "The number on the scale or on the clothing label does not determine my worth. It took my husband's and my daughters' love to teach me that."

She still monitors her weight and how her clothes fit. "But they do not determine my mood," she says. "I use them like I use a speedometer in a car. There is a place I'd like to be, and they are a tool to help me stay within a range and make minor adjustments as necessary."

THE TAKEAWAY

Make a good mix. Use measures you can take on a daily, weekly, and more long-term basis, plus measures that are affordable and easy to access. And think beyond the numbers. Remember, your overall health and happiness matters more than anything. If your heart, lungs, romance, or job is breaking down, your running and weight-loss goals won't mean much.

Give it 4 weeks. Remember, as George Sheehan once said, you're an experiment of one. Try this mix for at least 4 weeks to see if it works for you. If after that time you're feeling like you're not getting the feedback you're seeking, then switch it up.

Make it personal. Regardless of the science, or our recommendations, only you can decide what matters most to you.

A NOTE ON DISORDERED EATING

Reaching for your weight-loss and racing goals takes a tremendous amount of focus and effort. Making radical changes to what you eat, how you eat, and how you work out can feel downright consuming.

Even before you take a step or digest a single calorie, you can end up spending a lot of time and attention doing research, planning out what you'll eat and where you'll buy it, deciding what you'll order at restaurants, and standing in the grocery aisles scrutinizing food labels to assess whether, given a food's calorie, sugar, protein, and nutrient content, it deserves a place on your plate. It can be overwhelming, especially if you've never watched what you've eaten before.

Jarring as it can be, it does get easier with practice. In this book, you get a heaping helping of information about how to design your Run to Lose diet to include the healthiest and most delicious foods that will energize you and help you run your best. In short order, information will morph into knowledge. Over time, knowledge will morph into understanding. And eventually, once you find the right mix of healthy foods that helps you feel and run your best, choosing healthy foods becomes second nature.

But if your friends, colleagues, and loved ones are not watching what they eat, your newfound commitment to nutrition may seem abrupt to them and may require some adjustment. They may accuse you of being "obsessed" or even of having an eating disorder.

While they will adjust to your new healthy habits just as you will, as you embark on this journey, it's important to understand when a healthy commitment to weight-loss goals crosses the line into an unhealthy, disordered relationship with food and weight.

Where is that line? "It's not a simple answer," says Riley Nickols, PhD, clinical coordinator at the Victory Program at McCallum Place Eating Disorders Treatment Program in St. Louis, Missouri. The Victory

Program specializes in treating elite high school and adult athletes with eating disorders.

Disordered eating isn't just about a newfound scrutiny over calories and nutrients. Eating disorders—including anorexia, bulimia, and binge eating disorder—are serious problems that require medical attention right away. "Eating disorders are very similar to alcohol or substance abuse," says Nickols. "They negatively impact your social life, your work performance, and start to filter over to other parts of life."

You should watch out for some warning signs if you're concerned that you or a loved one has developed an eating disorder. They include:

- Repeated injuries due to low fat, carb, and protein intake
- Overwhelming guilt about taking days off from running
- Overly rigid, abnormal eating patterns and behaviors
- Lack of flexibility about what, when, and how much to eat
- Isolation and avoidance of eating in social situations
- Resistance to regaining weight to attain healthy weight
- Poor body image; certain body parts feel intolerable
- Body checking (repeatedly and obsessively grabbing or holding one part of the body)

"Normal eating incorporates a variety of foods, quantities, and eating at different times of days," says Nickols.

What's so difficult about disordered eating among athletes is that they tend to exhibit a lot of traits like commitment and discipline that are admired and applauded in anyone who is working doggedly toward a goal. But athletes with eating disorders "take the good traits to an absolute extreme," says Nickols.

While a runner with a newfound commitment to weight loss and racing might be willing to run in any weather condition, someone with an eating disorder might be willing to run with a stress fracture. One prominent feature of an eating disorder can "involve a total denial of discomfort," Nickols says.

Often those with eating disorders also struggle with anxiety and/or depression. For those with disordered eating patterns, certain physical signs and symptoms start to emerge. "Your body speaks to you all the time," says Nickols. "Whether you choose to listen to it is another question."

After periods of intense dieting and disordered eating, max VO_2 (aerobic power) plummets along with running performance. If you're severely restricting nutrients like carbs and protein, it will take longer to recover from workouts, and you put yourself at serious risk of injuries in bones, muscles, and joints. While overuse injuries are inherent to all runners to some extent, the risk is "really heightened when you're not fueling appropriately," Nickols says. "The body will only perform optimally if you take care of it and fuel it to meet your energy needs."

Nickols strongly recommends that anyone struggling with disordered eating should get treatment from trained therapists who specialize in eating disorders. And for anyone working on weight loss and racing, it's a good idea to work with a sports dietitian to understand how many calories and what kinds of nutrients you need to get fit without getting hurt, or getting sick.

"Treatment of an eating disorder entails a tremendous need to transform your relationship with your body and with food," says Nickols, "and reshape your relationship with exercise in order to be healthier and recover long term."

PART I

WHAT TO EAT

With the barrage of dieting advice grabbing the headlines, it's hard to keep up with exactly which foods are aiding your weight-loss efforts and which ingredients are dragging you down. One day saturated fats are the culprit for the obesity epidemic; the next day it's gluten. The next day we're reading that most fats are fine, but all carbs are the cause of our frustrations.

One thing is for certain: If you're running on a regular basis or training for a race, the rules regarding *what* to eat are different than they are for other people who are looking to lose weight. If you have endured the frustration of watching the numbers on the scale increase right along with your weekly mileage, you understand this. You need all food groups to shed weight and get faster. And you need different kinds of foods than the average, nonrunning dieter needs.

In Part I, you'll learn about the best carbs, fats, protein, drinks, and sports foods you can eat to shrink your waistline, improve your race times, and increase your chances of living a long and happy life. And there's good news. *Run to Lose* is not about deprivation or exercising saintly feats of restraint. In fact it's more than likely that, after reading this section, you'll discover you need to indulge in a lot more of some truly delicious foods in order to reach your goals.

CHAPTER

1

All about Carbs

Since the 1970s, carbs have gotten a bad rap, thanks in large part to the popularity of certain diet plans. They've been demonized as the culprits of everything from dementia to anxiety, not to mention the country's chronic weight-control issues.

To some extent, this is justified. With over 520 calories, 74 grams of carbs, and 44 grams of sugar, a large bakery blueberry muffin[1] isn't going to do you any favors. And yes, lots of runners tend to take the carb-loading too far, with the 2,000-calorie dishes of spaghetti the night before a 5-K.

But when it comes to carbs, quality counts a lot. There is a huge chasm between that blueberry muffin from the bakery, which contains lots of fats, calories, and sugars with little nutritional benefit, and high-quality carbs such as a banana, an apple, or a sprouted piece of bread. These also contain fiber and nutrients that provide the fuel you need to run well and take your fitness to the next level, and vital minerals that protect you from chronic disease.

As a runner, 55 to 65 percent of your daily calories should come from high-quality carbs. During times of heavy training and high mileage, aim for the high end of this range. If you're sidelined or when you're more focused on weight loss rather than high performance, aim for the lower end of the range. Since carbs are the most efficient fuel that the body can quickly absorb and process for energy, you'll want to include them daily.

CHEW ON THIS

The pressure to eliminate carbs altogether can be tempting. But runners need carbs like cars need gas. If you tried to go for a drive with an empty tank, you wouldn't get far. It's the same thing with running. Heading out for a workout on a tank empty of carbs is a waste of time.

Why Carbs Are Essential

Plenty of healthy carbs—fruits, vegetables, and whole grains—contain fiber, antioxidants, and a host of essential vitamins and minerals and deserve mainstay status in your daily diet, no matter what your weight-loss or racing goals are. Without carbs in your diet, you have no fuel or glycogen stores in your muscles. And without any fuel in the tank, it's going to be very, very difficult to get the maximum calorie burn out of your workout—or even get through a long run without bonking.

Carbs are simply the easiest form of calories for your body to convert to energy. It's just like fueling a car. If you're going on a long road trip—or trying to win the Indy 500—you want to fill up on the highest-octane fuel on the market.

Certainly some athletes have found that if their pace isn't intense and if they've worked at it, they can run on fat stores, but for most runners carbohydrates are essential. It is simply impossible to meet the energy requirements for high-intensity workouts such as speed sessions and endurance workouts such as long, slow distance runs when your diet is depleted of carbs.

Not only that, but carbs help keep you hydrated. (It's called a "carbohydrate" for a reason!) Water retention may not be music to your ears, but adequate hydration can help you run faster so that you burn more calories. And dehydration has been proven to make running at any pace feel harder.[2]

Not All Carbs Are Created Equal

Though you do need carbs, the type of carb you eat and when you eat it can have dramatically different effects on how you feel while you're on the road during your run and what you see on the bathroom scale.

You want to focus on getting the highest-quality carbs with the most nutrients and the fewest unhealthy additives. Look at the list below. Each serving contains approximately 25 grams of carbs. For a complete list of the healthiest carbs for you, see page 59 for a list of healthy whole grains and pages 46 to 48 for a table of fruits and vegetables that can help you meet your carbohydrate needs.

- Grains (2 slices whole wheat bread, or 1 cup oatmeal, or ½ cup rice)
- Dairy products (2 cups low-fat or fat-free milk, or one 4.5-ounce, fruit-flavored yogurt)
- Beans and starchy vegetables (½ cup black beans, or 1 cup green peas, or 1 medium potato)
- Sports drinks, bars, and gels (1 energy bar, or 2 cups sports drink, or 1 carbohydrate gel)
- Mixed dishes (¾ cup tomato soup, or 1 slice thin-crust pizza, or 1 small vegetarian burrito)
- Fruits and juices (1 medium apple, or 2 cups fresh strawberries, or ¾ cup orange juice)

How Many Carbs Do You Need Each Day?

How many carbs you need depends on how hard you're training and what stage of training you're in. The reason many runners fail to reach their weight-loss goals, or worse, actually gain weight when they start running regularly, is that they're consuming more carbs than their level of running really demands. While there's nothing wrong with a large plate of pasta the night before a long run or a celebratory bagel after a long, hard workout, when you're trying to lose weight, there's probably no need for these types of foods every day of the week.

For weight-conscious runners, meeting your goals will come down to getting the carbs you need to avoid hitting the wall, without stuffing yourself silly.

If you're not training for a race, aim for 2.2 grams of carbohydrate per pound of body weight per day. As you ramp up mileage and intensity, increase your intake to 3.2 to 4 grams per pound of body weight. If you're carb-loading a few days before a race (more on that in Chapter 20), aim for 4.5 to 5.5 grams of carbs per pound of body weight per day. Here are two general rules to follow when it comes to carbs.

1. **Tweak the formula.** Remember, these are recommendations. If you're getting tired—during daily activities or during your workouts—increase your intake a bit.

2. **Time it right.** Be sure to spread your intake over the course of the day to promote fuel availability for key training sessions— before, during, and after exercise. By consuming carbohydrate before, sometimes during, and after your workout (combined with protein) you'll feel energized during the run and ready to tackle future workouts without feeling overly fatigued and run-down. (See more on when to eat in Part III.)

THE TAKEAWAY

Count your daily carb needs. Try tracking your intake of carbs—rather than calories—for 1 week and see how it matches up to these recommendations. You may need to add more carbs, or reduce yours, to fuel your current running needs.

Add wholesome, high-quality carbs to your diet. If you've been eliminating them on a low-carb diet, try adding wholesome alternatives back for 1 week. Track how you feel on your runs and how quickly you recover for your next workout.

Time your carb intake right. Plan your meals so that you have your most carb-heavy meals and snacks immediately before, during, and right after hard workouts.

2

Fruits and Veggies: The Forlorn Fuel

The word *carb* summons dreamy visions of bagels, doughnuts, croissants, and an assortment of hot, steaming baked goods. But what many people—and many diets—overlook is that fresh fruits and vegetables actually provide a lot of the carbs any runner needs to rev up their workouts, without a lot of the additives and unsavory side effects that can weigh runners down on the road and on the scale.

Just compare a banana and a bagel—which runners often must choose between before a run or a race. From a cursory glance at the calorie count for each item, they seem roughly comparable. If anything, the bagel might seem like a slightly healthier choice. A small plain bagel has 180 calories, 36 grams of carb, 6 grams of sugar, and 7 grams of protein,[1] while one medium banana has 105 calories with 27 grams of carb, 14 grams of sugar, and 1.3 grams of protein. But look a little closer. The banana has a raft of other critical nutrients runners need—including vitamin B_6 (which helps convert proteins and sugars into energy and helps build cells), magnesium (which assists in muscle contractions and energy metabolism, endurance, and aerobic capacity), and potassium, which is critical to fending off electrolyte imbalances that can lead to muscle cramps on the run. The bagel has few to none of those special powers.

What's more, in recent years researchers have discovered the degree to which fresh produce can protect you from the most prevalent and menacing chronic diseases, like type 2 diabetes and cardiovascular disease.

That doesn't mean you have to become a vegetarian. But it does mean that whole fruits and vegetables can play a huge role in helping you have a long and healthy life, happily free of chronic diseases that have been accepted as part of aging for most of the American public. They can also provide a high-quality way to fuel up your runs.

Admittedly, bananas, apples, and carrots may not have the sensual appeal of a freshly baked bagel smothered with cream cheese, or even the sweet memories or associations that go along with it. But the truth is that fresh produce can fuel you just as well and provide important nutrients and minerals that will help you bounce back quickly from tough workouts and prevent chronic diseases such as stroke, heart disease, and high blood pressure. And if you can fend off those ills, you're more likely to reach your goals at the finish line and on the bathroom scale.

Some fruits and veggies are better than others for your running life. In general, fruits and vegetables you consume with the peel attached (such as apples and potatoes) and most berries will contain lots of fiber. Fiber is great, as it will keep you feeling full and help you fend off chronic disease.

CHEW ON THIS

When it comes to the benefits of fruits and veggies, your waistline and your workouts are just the tip of the iceberg. A 2012 study in the *European Journal of Nutrition* concluded that there's convincing evidence that fruits and veggies can reduce the risk of high blood pressure, heart disease, and stroke and may even lower risk of cancer, prevent weight gain associated with type 2 diabetes, and lower risk of eye diseases, dementia, osteoporosis, asthma, COPD, and rheumatoid arthritis.[2]

But if you're heading out the door for a run in the next 60 minutes, avoid any produce that has more than 7 grams of fiber per serving.

Below you'll find some of the highest-carb whole fruits and vegetables with extra nutrients that will support your running. It's best to eat what's in season whenever possible. When produce is harvested before its peak—say it's February, and red peppers have to be picked early in Mexico to meet the demand in Missouri—they don't contain the full supply of nutrients they would have if they had been harvested when they were ready. Plus, when produce is being shipped long distances, nutrients can be lost across the journey and preservatives are often added to protect it from spoilage during travel.

FUELING UP WITH FRUITS AND VEGGIES

FRUIT/ VEGGIE	CARBS (G)/ SERVING	FIBER (G)/ SERVING	EXTRA NUTRIENTS FOR RUNNERS
Banana (1 large)	31	4	Bananas contain potassium, B_6, and magnesium, which help maintain hydration on the run and fend off muscle cramps.
Figs, dried (1)	5	1	Figs are rich in carbs and potassium, and they're also easy to carry. Figs make a great midrun snack.
Sweet potato (1 medium)	27	4 (with skin)	Sweet potatoes are tasty and loaded with vitamin A, which is commonly known to improve eyesight.
Pear (1 medium)	27	5	Pears contain quercetin, a phytonutrient linked to preventing disease such as cancer as well as potentially improving athletic performance.
Cranberries, sweetened, dried (¼ cup)	25	2	Cranberries contain compounds called proanthocyanidins, which have been shown to prevent stomach ulcers, urinary tract infections, and cavities and improve cardiovascular health. Combine cranberries with other dried berries and you'll have an antioxidant-rich blend that can prevent inflammation.

FRUIT/ VEGGIE	CARBS (G)/ SERVING	FIBER (G)/ SERVING	EXTRA NUTRIENTS FOR RUNNERS
Butternut squash (½ cup cooked cubes)	11	3	A superb source of vitamin A, just one serving offers men 64% and women 82% of the recommended daily intake of this vision-supporting nutrient.
Cauliflower (½ cup raw)	3	1	Cauliflower contains vitamin C, folate, and vitamin B_6. Vitamin C boosts immunity, helps the body absorb iron, and helps the body create collagen, a critical component of every tendon, ligament, and connective tissue. Vitamin B_6 plays a critical role in metabolism. Folate helps the body process amino acids; it's important to get because it's lost in sweat, urine, and stool. If you're trying to cut calories, try mashed cauliflower, which has a look and texture similar to higher-calorie mashed potatoes.
Dates (1)	18	2	Like other dried fruits, dates are a portable source of energizing carb, so they make a great choice for refueling on the run. Dates are also rich in phosphorus, an electrolyte that plays a key role in maintaining fluid balance and is essential for healthy bones.
Raisins (1 box/1.5 oz)	34	2	Easily digestible, portable, and energy dense, raisins are a great on-the-go fueling option. They also contain quite a bit of potassium and other electrolytes such as magnesium, calcium, and sodium.
Kiwi (1)	10	2	This fruit is rich in tissue-repairing vitamin C.
Navel orange (1 medium)	18	3	While an obvious choice for vitamin C to boost your immunity, an orange also contains carbs and fluids to help you stay energized and hydrated.
Strawberries, whole (1 cup)	11	3	Put more strawberries on your plate and you'll get more vitamin C in your body. Strawberries contain anthocyanins, which can help repair muscles and fight inflammation.
Carrots, baby (10)	8	3	Eating carrots is one of the best ways to receive your Daily Value of vitamin A, and the orange vegetable also has vitamin B_6 and carotene to give your immune system a boost.

(continued)

FUELING UP WITH FRUITS AND VEGGIES (CONT.)

FRUIT/ VEGGIE	CARBS (G)/ SERVING	FIBER (G)/ SERVING	EXTRA NUTRIENTS FOR RUNNERS
Spaghetti squash (½ cup cooked)	5	1	Compared to "real" pasta, spaghetti squash offers more nutrients as well as filling fiber. If you're counting calories, spaghetti squash is ideal because copious amounts of this easy-to-prepare vegetable contain just a handful of calories. Served with pasta sauce and cheese, it's a great guilt-free alternative to pasta.
Blackberries (½ cup)	7	4	Low in calories and high in antioxidants, blackberries contain fiber and vitamin C, plus vitamin K, which strengthens bones.
Blueberries (½ cup)	10	2	Blueberries contain powerful phytochemicals and antioxidants that may reduce risk of various cancers and heart disease while working to fight inflammation. Research is now under way to understand how the phytochemicals in blueberries could improve brain function.
Tomato (½ cup chopped)	4	1	Tomatoes are strong sources of vitamin C, vitamin K, and vitamin A, plus potassium, which can aid in recovery from tough workouts.
Grapefruit (½ large)	13	2	Grapefruit offers healthy doses of vitamin C, potassium, and folate. Potassium can help keep your muscles from cramping. Red grapefruits have the same amount of vitamin C as white grapefruits, plus vitamin A and pantothenic acid, which your body uses to transform proteins, fats, and carbohydrates into energy.
Cabbage (1 cup cooked)	8	3	Cabbage is a leafy green that is low in calories, has high concentrations of vitamins K and C, and is a good source of folate. Runners can protect the health of red blood cells by increasing their intake of folate.
Yams (½ cup cooked cubes)	19	3	Like sweet potatoes, yams can be mashed and taken on the run for a natural fueling option. A sprinkle of salt combined with the 456 mg of naturally present potassium makes a great midrun fuel option.
Grapes (1 cup)	16	1	Like the wine that is made from them, red and purple grapes contain the rare antioxidant resveratrol, which is linked to a healthier heart.

Not All Produce Is Created Equal

Fruits have gotten a bit of a bad name in recent years, as low-carb diets have become more popular and researchers have learned more about the dangers of sugar. Yes, fruits contain naturally occurring sugar, but the 23 grams of naturally occurring sugar in an orange are not going to wreak the same havoc on your body as the same amount of added sugar in, say, a doughnut. Why? In addition to sugar, fruits have important vitamins, minerals, and phytonutrients to stave off chronic disease and keep you healthy, plus water to keep you hydrated. What's more, the fiber in the skins of fruits and veggies means that they are digested more gradually, so they don't cause the same kinds of energy spikes and crashes as table sugar. And the fiber boosts heart health and keeps your GI system working efficiently. If you're looking to reduce the amount of sugar in your diet, cut out the processed foods with added sugars; keep the fruit, which has so many other nutrients that are critical for good health.

That said, not all fruits and veggies are created equal. Almost always, eating produce in its raw form is your best bet. One cup of dried apple pieces, for example, can have 49 grams of sugar and 209 calories and will likely leave you hungry. That same cup of raw apples will have just 57 calories and 13 grams of sugar, plus water, fiber, and other essential vitamins and nutrients. Even dried veggies can be full of added sugars, fat, and sodium that you don't need. Packaged products such as kale chips, beet chips, or freeze-dried sugar snap peas may seem like healthier alternatives. But take a look at the ingredient list and Nutrition Facts, and you'll see that many of these products rival potato chips in terms of calories and fat. If you want something to satisfy a crunchy, salty craving, your best bet is to make your own.

The Best of the Best

Which fruits and veggies are the healthiest? In 2014, researchers from the Centers for Disease Control and Prevention attempted to rank them according to their nutrient density. These so-called produce powerhouses, created by Jennifer Di Noia, PhD, of William Paterson University in New Jersey, are found to reduce heart disease and some cancers. The list ranks 47 foods according to their density of 17 nutrients including iron, riboflavin, niacin, folate, vitamin B_6, vitamin B_{12}, vitamin C, and vitamin K.[3]

Topping the list was watercress, a leafy green packed full of antioxidants and vitamin K, followed by Chinese cabbage, chard, beet greens, spinach, chicory, leaf lettuce, parsley, romaine lettuce, collard greens, turnip greens, mustard greens, endive, chives, kale, dandelion greens, red pepper, arugula, broccoli, pumpkin, Brussels sprouts, scallions, kohlrabi, cauliflower, cabbage, and carrots.

Better Together

Some foods can accentuate the nutrients in other foods. This is often referred to as food synergy. Here are some foods that bring out the best in one another.

Vitamin D + calcium: Vitamin D helps the body absorb calcium, which you need to build strong bones and stave off stress fractures. The Institute of Medicine recommends that most adults get 600 IU of vitamin D and 1,000 milligrams of calcium every day.

Serving suggestion: Get calcium from dairy products such as milk, cheese, and yogurt and broccoli, kale, and Chinese cabbage. Some foods, such as oatmeal, orange juice, and cereal, are fortified with calcium. Vitamin D can come from salmon, tuna, sardines, mackerel, shrimp, mushrooms, egg yolks, and fortified items such as select orange juices and breads.

Iron + vitamin C: In addition to boosting immunity so you don't get sidelined by coughs and colds, vitamin C helps the body absorb iron. That's especially important if you're a vegetarian and rely on plant-based sources of iron (which aren't absorbed as readily) such as lentils, chickpeas, and black beans.

Serving suggestion: Good sources of vitamin C include tomato, broccoli, citrus fruits, leafy greens, strawberries, bell peppers, and broccoli. Iron can be found in beet greens, kale, spinach, mustard seeds, and fortified cereal.

Veggies + healthy fats: Monounsaturated fats—such as those in olive oil, avocado, walnuts, and almonds—not only help lower cholesterol and reduce heart disease risk but also help the body absorb antioxidants and essential fat-soluble vitamins—such as A,D, E, and K—from veggies including carrots, broccoli, peas, spinach, and sweet potatoes.

Serving suggestion: Top your salad with a serving of full-fat dressing, walnuts, pistachios, or grated cheese. Add olive oil to your favorite pasta with marinara dish.

Protein + carbs: Protein not only builds muscle and helps fill you up but also slows the absorption of sugar from carbs into your body so you're less likely to have cravings. When you do eat healthy carbs from whole grains, fruits, and veggies, pair them with protein. This is especially important if you're refueling postrun. Research has shown that having a protein-and-carb snack in the 30 to 60 minutes following a workout (see Chapter 22 on eating for recovery) can help you bounce back quickly for your next run.

Serving suggestion: Cereal topped with milk or graham crackers spread with peanut butter contain both carbs and protein. Try apples with cashew butter or a pita filled with hummus. Or try tuna fish mixed with honey mustard on whole grain bread.

Preserving the Nutrients on the Way to Your Plate

All those nutrient-packed fruits and veggies won't do you any good if, on the way to your plate, you kill all the nutrients in the cooking process. Many vitamins—including water-soluble vitamins such as

C, thiamin, riboflavin, folate, and B$_{12}$—are sensitive to heat, air, and, in the case of riboflavin, even light exposure. In general, the longer you cook produce, the more water you use, and the higher the temperature, the more nutrients (and taste) you'll lose. Here are some tips on how you can preserve the healing powers—and the flavor— of produce.

Go raw. In most cases, you can't go wrong consuming whole produce in its natural state in salads, smoothies, or as a stand-alone snack.

Be a minimalist. Keep the cooking time, temperature, and the amount of water needed to a minimum. Water leaches water-soluble vitamins from the food. Don't believe it? When you're finished cooking your veggies, take a look at the water. If it's colorful, those are the water-soluble vitamins that have been washed away. If you want to save them, you could drink the water or use it as a vegetable stock.

Steam it. A steamer—a colander with holes that you put over a pot of boiling water—cooks the veggies quickly so you can preserve valuable nutrients. It's the best way to preserve antioxidants in broccoli and zucchini.

Boil it. Boiling occurs at a high temperature, and the water can wash away vitamins and minerals in certain veggies. If you're boiling, keep the pot covered so you can cook the food quickly and expose it to high temperatures for as short a time as possible. And use the leftover water—which will be packed with nutrients from your veggies—in sauces and soups.

Zap it. Microwaves have gotten a bad rap—"nuking" your food has been associated with fears about radiation. But scores of trials have established that they're perfectly safe. Cooks also know that the high zap allows you to keep cooking time brief and use little water.

Stir-fry it. Cooking your vegetables over high heat in a small amount of oil for a short amount of time can minimize nutrient loss and is a tasty way to prepare meat, rice, and julienned veggies.

Grill it. This method allows you to cook with minimal added fats, while preserving the flavor and the juiciness. While there's limited conclusive evidence, some research suggests regularly eating charred, well-done meat can increase risk of some cancers. When you are barbecuing, stick with lean cuts and smaller portions that you won't have to cook as long. With lean cuts there's less fat to drip down and create flare-ups. And consider using a marinade; according to the American Institute for Cancer Research, studies have shown that by marinating your meat before grilling, you can potentially decrease the formation of carcinogenic compounds by up to 96 percent, possibly thanks to the antioxidants that are present in the marinade.[4]

Try baking or roasting. This method helps some vegetables retain, and even boost, their nutrients. That includes artichokes, asparagus, broccoli, green beans, eggplant, corn, Swiss chard, spinach, and peppers. Other veggies lose their antioxidant power when exposed to high heat. These include Brussels sprouts, leeks, cauliflower, peas, zucchini, onions, beans, celery, beets, and garlic. So either bake them quickly, blanch (don't boil) them, or consider eating them raw whenever possible.

Try juicing. Juicing and making smoothies can be a great way to get raw fruits and veggies into your diet, as long as you keep the drinks full of healthy things. Sometimes these drinks can be calorie bombs that rival the nutrition content of milkshakes. While juicing can have some health benefits, especially for those who weren't incorporating produce into their diets before, the juicing process that some juicers and extractors use does take away the nutritious pulp and fiber produce contains, so you'll need to find sources of fiber elsewhere. If you're looking for a smoothie or shake that doesn't derail your daily calorie target, use whole fruits and veggies (frozen varieties are fine). Avoid adding honey, fruit juice concentrate, sweetened yogurt, whole milk, cream, or even ice cream. The most powerful smoothies should contain at least two servings of fruits and veggies. If you're looking to make your smoothie into a recovery drink, be sure to include a source of protein such as 100 percent whey protein powder, fat-free milk, or Greek yogurt. (For more on juicing diets, see page 139.)

THE TAKEAWAY

Assess your fruit and veggie intake. Think about your regular meals and snacks. How many fruits and veggies are you getting on a regular basis? Be sure to get the timing right. If you're headed out the door for a run within the next 60 minutes, avoid any produce that has more than 7 grams of fiber per serving.

Add a serving of veggies to one meal every day. Can't stand veggies? Grind them up and add them to your marinara sauce. Toss them in the blender with ice, yogurt, and milk for smoothies.

Add a serving of fruit as a snack. Bananas, oranges, apples, and other fruits make great portable, filling, and satisfying snacks you can take with you when you're on the go.

CHAPTER

3

Good Grains

With the uproar over carbs in recent years, grains have unfortunately gotten a bad reputation they don't deserve. Grains have been blamed for obesity and weight problems; many runners, dieters, and celebrities advocate eliminating them to reach your feel-great weight.

But just as with sugars, there's a huge difference between the refined grains in products such as crackers, cookies, rolls, and doughnuts, which really are the culprits behind many people's weight problems, and the whole grains in foods such as oats, buckwheat, quinoa, and wild rice, which have real health benefits.

While refined grains can be hazardous to your diet, whole grains are an essential part of it. Try to eliminate whole grains altogether, and you'll have a tough time reaching your weight-loss and racing goals.

In this chapter, you'll learn why whole grains are such an important part of your diet and how to distinguish them from the more troublesome refined grains that can derail your goals.

Whole Grains versus Refined Grains

Whole grains include the endosperm, germ, and bran, in the same proportions as when they were harvested from the earth. Rich in antioxidants and nutrients, whole grains have been shown to lower blood pressure and cholesterol; reduce risk of cancer, heart disease, type 2 diabetes, and obesity; and thanks to their higher fiber content, even improve glucose and insulin response to a meal. A study in the January 2015 issue of the *Journal of the American Medical Association* linked a diet rich in whole grains with a significantly lower risk of death from heart disease.[1]

And contrary to the widely held carb-o-phobia that has taken hold in recent years, there's also evidence that whole grains *can* help you reach your weight-loss goals. A study published in the January 2008 issue of the *American Journal of Clinical Nutrition* found that individuals who consumed a diet rich in whole grains had less belly fat and a smaller waist circumference than individuals who reached for the white bread.[2] The high fiber content of whole grains helps you feel fuller longer, which can help prevent overeating.

While refined grains—the kind found in white bread, traditional pastas, cookies, doughnuts, and croissants—will energize you for your runs, they don't have the same long-term health benefits. Refined grains have been stripped of the nutrient-rich bran, germ, and endosperm—often for the sake of taste, texture, and a longer shelf life at the grocery store.

In fact, these items often have a lot of saturated fats, sugar, sodium, and empty calories that can keep you from reaching your weight-loss goals. Plus, they can wreak havoc with your blood sugar. They tend to

CHEW ON THIS

How do you tell if a product contains whole grains? Many, but not all, products carry a Whole Grain stamp on the food label. If you don't see the stamp, scan the ingredient list. If it includes ingredients containing the word *whole* as the first (few) ingredient(s), you can safely assume it's a whole grain. Other terms, such as *unbleached* and *stone ground*, may sound fancy but typically mean the grain is refined.

lack fiber and they don't offer the same fullness benefits that whole grains provide. Because they're digested so quickly, they cause the blood sugar to spike then quickly plummet, leaving you feeling depleted.

Since research links chronic diseases, such as diabetes and heart disease, to diets that send your blood sugar on a roller-coaster ride, it's best to avoid refined, highly processed grains.

Whole grains provide a steady, slow release of energy. Most whole grains score low on the glycemic index (read more about that in Chapter 5). Whole grain barley, for instance, has a GI score of 25, while white baguette has a GI of 95.

How Much Whole Grain Do You Need?

Because whole grains are a carbohydrate, the amount you should target depends, to some degree, on how hard you're training and what your weight-loss goals are. The more intense your workouts, the more whole grains you'll need. (For more information on how much carbohydrate to aim for each day, see Chapter 1.) That said, most people need to ratchet up their whole grain intake, no matter how hard they're training. The 2010 Dietary Guidelines recommend that most adults eat *at least* three to five servings of whole grains every day. At least half the grains you consume should be whole grains.

Getting the Timing Right

The key to working whole grains into your diet—without derailing your racing and weight-loss goals—is to make sure you're getting the right amounts at the right time.

Whole grains do pack a calorie punch, and because foods such as rice, oatmeal, and cereal are easy to overeat, it's important to measure out your portions. Here are some examples of single servings of popular whole grain items.

- $\frac{1}{2}$ cup cooked rice, bulgur, pasta, or cereal
- 1 ounce dry pasta, rice, or other dry grain
- 1 slice bread
- 1 small muffin (weighing 1 ounce)
- 1 cup ready-to-eat cereal flakes

Because of the high-fiber nature of whole grains, it's important to time your intake right. Downing a piece of whole grain bread immediately prerun can lead to GI distress. To prevent a midrun pit stop, your prerun meal should have less than 7 grams of fiber.

It's best to save whole grains for a postworkout meal, when your body is primed to absorb the nutrients, repair muscle, and restock spent glycogen stores. (Read more about eating for recovery in Chapter 22.)

Any whole grain foods make an ideal postrun meal, because they also contain protein and amino acids, which can fire up the recovery process. Top a slice of whole wheat toast with a scrambled egg, toss some wheat berries with spinach and grilled chicken breast, add some edamame to a bowl of brown rice, or enjoy a fat-free latte with your morning whole grain bagel.

Finding the Highest-Quality Whole Grains for You

With flashy packaging and caramel coloring, it can be difficult to tell a refined grain from a true whole grain. Not all brown or wheat breads have whole grains. And now there are even some white whole-grain breads.

The quickest way to spot whole grain is to look for the Whole Grain

HEALTHY WHOLE GRAINS

GRAIN	EXTRA BENEFITS FOR RUNNERS
Amaranth	Amaranth is rich in protein as well as minerals such as calcium, iron, magnesium, and phosphorus. These promote strong bones and healthy blood but these nutrients are often limited in the average diet.
Barley	With 8 grams of fiber in a ¼-cup serving, barley offers more fiber than any other whole grain. It's also high in antioxidants, vitamins, and minerals, such as magnesium and phosphorus, which are needed for bone health, plus iron and potassium, which are needed for healthy blood and circulation. Be sure to buy whole grain or hulled barley; pearled barley is missing at least some of the bran layer.
Buckwheat	A popular ingredient in pancake mixes, soba noodles, kasha, and other foods, buckwheat contains higher levels of zinc, copper, and manganese, essential nutrients that are needed in small amounts but can be hard to find in the average diet. Buckwheat also has a high level of muscle-boosting protein, about 6 grams in 1 cup of cooked groats. It's also high in soluble fiber (to improve cholesterol levels) and resistant starch (to improve digestive health).
Corn	Corn provides more than 10 times as much vision-boosting vitamin A as other grains. Corn is also high in antioxidants and carotenoids that are associated with eye health. And because it's gluten-free, corn is popular with those who have celiac disease or follow a gluten-free diet.
Oats	If you see *oats* or *oat flour* on the label, you can be sure you're getting whole grain. Oats almost never have their bran and germ removed in processing. Oats have been widely studied and linked with reduced risk of heart disease, type 2 diabetes, some cancers, and even asthma. And for the weight-conscious runner they're ideal; 1 cup of cooked oats has about 6 grams of protein (more if you make your morning oats with milk rather than water) and roughly 2 grams of heart-healthy unsaturated fat per serving, more than most other grains. That fat will help keep you feeling fuller longer.
Quinoa	Because it's gluten-free and is one of the few grains that provide a complete protein, quinoa has never been more popular. Easy to cook and ready in about 15 minutes, it's a popular choice for vegetarians, both on its own and as an ingredient in energy bars, shakes, cereals, and other health foods. With 159 milligrams of potassium in a ½-cup serving, quinoa has more potassium than other whole grains. Potassium helps fight muscle cramps and lower blood pressure.
Rice (brown, black, red, or others)	Easy to cook and easy to tolerate, rice is an excellent source of carbs for a postrun recovery meal. Most whole grain varieties are high in fiber and nutrients such as manganese and selenium, which is important for carbohydrate and fat metabolism.
Rye	Rye has a high amount of fiber in its endosperm—not just in its bran. Because of this, products made with rye generally have a lower glycemic index than products made from other whole grains. Rye contains a unique type of dietary fiber, arabinoxylan, known for its high antioxidant activity, which helps fight inflammation to ease muscle soreness. Research has shown that rye boosts GI health and leads to satiety, so you can stay fuller longer, which can help you manage your weight.
Whole wheat	By far the most common grain used in breads, pastas, and other foods, whole wheat has been shown to reduce risk of stroke, type 2 diabetes, heart disease, overweight, asthma, inflammatory disease, and other illnesses.
Wild rice	When compared to other types of rice—like brown rice—wild rice has twice the protein and fiber but less iron and calcium.

emblem of the Whole Grain Council. If the label has that emblem, it will also likely say how much whole grain the food contains. The stamp guarantees that the product provides at least 8 grams of whole grain per serving. If you don't see an emblem, look for the word *whole* before grains in the list of ingredients. For more info on whole grains, one of the best resources to check out is the Whole Grains Council (wholegrainscouncil.org).

See page 59 for a list of some of the best whole grains for runners and the extra health benefits they provide.

Gluten-Free Grains

Staying away from gluten? That doesn't mean you have to go grain-free. A variety of gluten-free grains are on the market.[3] They include:

- Amaranth
- Buckwheat
- Corn
- Millet
- Montina
- Oats
- Quinoa
- Rice
- Sorghum
- Teff
- Wild rice

THE TAKEAWAY

Make simple swaps. To get your three to five servings of whole grains each day, cut back the number of products with refined grains, such as white rolls, butter crackers, and others. Increase the number made from whole wheat, whole grain corn, brown rice, steel-cut oats, and quinoa.

Read the list of ingredients. Look for the Whole Grain emblem on food packages as well as the word *whole* on the ingredient panel (not just *wheat*). Remember, just because a bread is brown in color doesn't mean it contains whole grains.

Time your intake right. Avoid consuming whole grains right before a run, because they take longer to digest, and that could lead to GI distress. Make whole grains a part of regular meals and consume them immediately after a hard workout—like a long run or speedwork—when the body needs carbs to restock spent glycogen stores and repair muscles, so you can bounce back for the next workout.

4

Getting Smart about Sugar

Sugar is a diet demon that's earned its bad rap. Overloading on sugar can lead to lots of unwanted pounds and a wide range of health problems, including heart disease, diabetes, and high blood pressure.

In the last few decades, the dangers of excessive sugar intake have been well documented. If you need motivation to stay away from the sweet stuff, consider this research.

It can lead to diabetes. A constant intake of sugar forces your pancreas to work overtime, possibly leading to type 2 diabetes down the road. It also lowers levels of HDL (good) cholesterol while increasing triglycerides. Both increase the risk of heart disease.[1]

It can lead to other chronic diseases. In a February 2012 study published in *Nature*, researchers pointed out that too much sugar leads to obesity; damages the liver and metabolism; impairs brain function; and increases risk of heart disease and cancer.[2]

It makes you hungry. Overdosing on sugar sends your hunger hormones into overdrive. The satiety hormones that tell your brain "I'm full!" aren't properly triggered, which means you end up eating more than you need to.

It's as addictive as drugs. And since it's legal, maybe more so. In addition to having all these toxic effects on your health, sugar gives you a rush that makes you want more. If you've ever tried to eat just one square of milk chocolate, you've likely discovered there's no satisfying a sweet tooth. In a July 2013 study published in the journal *Current Opinion in Clinical Nutrition and Metabolic Care*,[3] researchers concluded that "evidence in humans shows that sugar and sweetness can induce reward and craving that are comparable in magnitude to those induced by addictive drugs." While it's difficult to compare the different rewards of a sugar high from one you might get from a drug like cocaine, in experiments on lab rats, the researchers showed that sugar and sweet rewards "can not only substitute to addictive drugs, like cocaine, but can even be more rewarding and attractive."

With all these dire warnings about sugar, it's tempting to reach for calorie-free artificial sweeteners when you want a treat. But many

CHEW ON THIS

On packaged foods, the Nutrition Facts label will show how many grams of sugar per serving the product contains. Although you can't always isolate the natural sugars from added sugars—they're all lumped together in *total* sugars—there are ways to tell if a product is high in dangerous added sugars. If the product has no fruit or milk products in the ingredients, all the sugars in the food are from added sugars. If the product contains fruit or milk products, the total sugar per serving listed on the label will include added and naturally occurring sugars.

Unless you're consuming a fruit or dairy product, in general it's best to aim for less than 10 grams of sugar per serving, or one that provides less than 5 percent of the recommended Daily Value (which will be shown as "%RDV" on the package). Anything that provides 20 percent or more of the recommended Daily Value is high in sugar. Keep in mind that 4 grams of sugar equals about 1 teaspoon, or 16 calories. So a 12-ounce can of regular cola might have 40 grams of sugar or 10 teaspoons of sugar. The American Heart Association recommends that women have no more than 6 teaspoons of sugar per day; men should have no more than 9 teaspoons per day.

people report that these sweeteners can drive up cravings for sweet stuff too. (Read more in Chapter 11 on sugar substitutes.)

Why Sugar from Fruits and Dairy Is Different

Many low-carb and high-protein diets discourage consumption of the natural sugars found in fruit, dairy products, and some starchy veggies (such as corn, peas, potatoes, baked beans, and more). But cutting out these fruits and veggies for the sake of cutting back on sugar would be a big mistake. The naturally occurring sugar in plain yogurt, a veggie, or a piece of fruit is much healthier than the added sugar in, say, a candy bar, because it's packaged with the vitamins and minerals you need to run strong, lose weight, and fend off chronic disease.

For instance, bananas contain sugar, but they also contain potassium, which helps prevent muscle cramping on the road. Raisins have fiber and iron; oranges have vitamin C to help fend off coughs and colds; and corn contains lutein, a vision-boosting nutrient that few other foods have. Carrots are high in vitamin A, which helps eyesight. And while milk contains lactose, a naturally occurring sugar, it also has bone-building calcium and vitamin D you need to stay strong.

Just take an apple and a candy bar, urges Dee McCaffrey, author of *The Science of Skinny*. The apple has "the perfect package of vitamins, fiber, enzymes, and phytonutrients," says McCaffrey, a chemist who lost more than 100 pounds by eliminating processed foods and starting a regular exercise regimen.

"When you eat the apple, it actually cleanses your body and your liver, the body's main fat-burning organ and the main filter of the body. When you eat something like an apple, it actually supports your whole metabolism and the detoxification pathways and fat burning," she says. "It's a very efficient form of calories that your body will use up and not store."

In contrast, when you eat 100 calories of a candy bar, you'll get fast energy, but you'll also get a lot of sugar, and you'll miss out on the cleansing, fat-burning, and general health benefits that you'd get from the apple. What's more, the refined sugar is inflammatory to the body.

"Even though you might get a burst of energy from eating that sugar, the candy bar could leave undetected chronic inflammation in the body and the arteries," McCaffrey says. "So the candy bar calories could be causing a long-term health issue. The apple is giving you a long-term health benefit."

Regardless of your daily calorie target, it's important to make room in your diet for whole, unprocessed fruits and starchy vegetables. Because fruits and veggies contain fiber and dairy products contain fat and protein, they won't make your blood sugar soar then crash the way the sugars in processed foods will. And the health benefits they provide vastly outweigh the fact that they have sugars.

How Much Sugar Should You Have?

You want to consume as little added sugar as possible. The American Heart Association advises women to limit added sugar to 100 calories or 25 grams per day; men should have no more than 150 calories or 27.5 grams per day. That said, it's nearly impossible to determine how much sugar in a packaged product is "added sugar" (from unhealthy additives) and how much of the sugar comes from natural sources such as fruits and dairy.

To make it simple, try to keep it under 10 grams of sugar per serving and don't stress out about amounts of sugar in raw fruits or milk. To stabilize your energy levels, try to consume this at even intervals throughout the day.

How to Avoid Sugar

Even if you avoid obvious sugar shocks you may still be consuming a lot of sugar that you don't need in your meals and snacks. Here's how to avoid sneaky sources of sugar.

- **Avoid added sugar.** Look for brands that clearly state on the label that there's "no added sugar." Often sugar is added to sauces and dressings to bolster taste when other substances such as fat are taken out.

- **Check the ingredients.** Ingredients are listed by weight, so the ingredients listed first make up a larger percentage of the product. If sugar (or another form of sugar included in the following list) is one of the first three ingredients, put it back.

- **Check the claims.** Packaged-foods manufacturers make a variety of claims about sugar content. Some of those claims have standard definitions. Others do not.

  - **Sugar-free:** Less than 0.5 gram of sugar per serving.

  - **Reduced sugar** or **less sugar:** At least 25 percent less sugar per serving compared to a standard serving size of the traditional variety.

  - **No added sugars** or **without added sugars:** This does not necessarily mean that the product is sugar-free. It just means that no sugars or no sugar-containing ingredients such as juice or dry fruit have been added. Any sugars in the product occur naturally.

  - **Low sugar:** There is no standard definition for this term. Be sure to check the Nutrition Facts panel on this one. The manufacturer may not define *low* the same way you do. (To read more on decoding food labels, turn to Chapter 12.)

- **Know sugar's other names.** Sugar is added to products in many different forms, but all of them offer calories and the same ill effects of sugar without any nutritional benefit. The following is a list of other forms of sugar you should look out for.

- Brown sugar
- Cane sugar
- Corn sugar
- Corn syrup
- Dextrose
- Fruit juice concentrate
- High fructose corn syrup

- Honey
- Maltodextrin
- Maltose
- Molasses
- Raw sugar
- Sucrose
- Turbinado sugar

Kyle's Story: Bagging Processed Foods

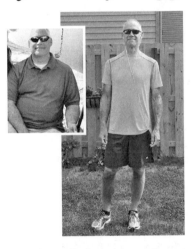

KYLE KLAVER, a 48-year-old sales engineer from Charlotte, North Carolina, was on a regular diet of convenience and fast foods, eating whatever was cheap and easy. That meant ready-to-make potatoes, frozen meals, bacon and sausage cooked in butter for breakfast, and fast food.

"It all has great taste," he says. But when he went to donate blood and was turned down due to high blood pressure, he started running in March 2014 with the help of a couch-to-5-K app. He started counting calories with a calorie-tracking app. For him, the key to losing 75 pounds and 10 pants sizes, and getting his blood pressure down to healthy levels, required much more than a 4-day-a-week running routine. The real game changer was eliminating processed foods.

"If it comes in a box or a bag, I won't eat it," he says. "We realized these types of foods are loaded with sodium, preservatives, and shelf stabilizers that have a lot of unknowns. These unknowns left us truly not knowing what we were eating."

At home he ate whole, fresh food with limited oils and butter. Invaluable, he says, was the support from his wife—who figured out how to reduce fat and sugar from everyday snacks and meals to make them healthy so he wouldn't feel deprived. "I wouldn't have been able to do this without her," he says. She got a boost too, and lost 50 pounds.

Kyle went from snacking on gummy worms, ice cream, chocolate candy, and chips to having fruit for dessert and snacking on nuts.

When traveling for work, which he does often, he started scouting out restaurants with healthy options ahead of time online. He became comfortable deconstructing any menu item to consume only the ingredients he wants to put in his body.

"Sometimes the restaurant will allow me to order a dish the way I want," he says. "Or I just order the standard and tear it apart at the table."

THE TAKEAWAY

Take stock of your daily sugar habits. Look at your average daily intake and calculate how much sugar you take in on a regular basis. Where can you cut out sugar? Try a 3-day detox from added sugars. Before you start, stock up on three different pieces of raw fruit that you enjoy. During the detox, anytime you crave a sweet, rather than trying to wrestle your own willpower to the ground, have a piece of fruit. At the end of 3 days, reassess how you feel and whether you miss anything you have taken out.

Don't drink it. Avoid any drinks with sugar, including sports drinks (unless you're on the run) and dressed-up coffee drinks. These won't fill you up the way foods do, nor do they offer any nutrition.

Set a standard for yourself. Avoid packaged foods with more than 10 grams of sugar per serving or foods that list sugar (in any form) in the first three ingredients.

CHAPTER 5

The Glycemic Index

If you've been searching for weight-loss guidance in recent years, it's likely you've heard about the glycemic index (GI). The index, which ranks foods according to how they affect your blood sugar, is designed to help you avoid foods that cause big swings in blood sugar that can lead to cravings, energy crashes, and chronic diseases such as type 2 diabetes. By the same token, the index can help you identify foods that will help you feel fuller longer.

The index assigns scores to different foods based on how quickly they're digested and enter the bloodstream and how much they make your blood sugar spike.

High-glycemic foods, such as bagels, pasta, and white bread, are ranked at 70 or higher, as they cause blood sugar to rise quickly. Lower-GI foods—such as fruits or old-fashioned oats—tend to be higher in fiber, protein, and fat; are slower to digest and absorb; and produce more gradual rises in blood sugar and insulin levels.

For the purpose of managing your weight, timing is everything when using the glycemic index. The high-GI foods may be ideal for giving you the burst of energy to power through that speed workout. But if you're constantly loading up on high-GI foods for sedentary activities such as a day at the office, it can be a problem. Why is that? Once your blood sugar rises, your body produces insulin to shuttle it back into the organs that need it. Too much of that over time can lead to chronic disease. And once your blood sugar falls, your energy level plummets, leading you to feel tired and hungry.

Like so many other factors, used in isolation, the glycemic index isn't a magic bullet that's going to catapult you to the PR of your dreams or get you to your feel-great weight. But used with all the other nutrition data you're gathering, it can help you tailor your diet to your racing and weight-loss goals.

How to Use GI to Reduce Finish Times and Your Waistline

While there is a fair amount of research looking at performance when fueling with a low- or high-GI diet, there is no solid answer as to how runners or dieters can use the GI best.

Some research shows that runners benefit from low-GI foods, as they provide a slow, steady supply of energy rather than cause you to crash and burn. In other words, you'll burn fat while saving the fuel that's in muscles and be able to run a bit longer before needing to pause for a snack. A study published in the July 2001 issue of the journal *Metabolism* concluded that when a moderate-GI carb was given to cyclists 45 minutes before exercise (in this case, rolled oats), they had more long-lasting energy than with higher-glycemic food (puffed rice).[1]

On the other hand, a study published in the November 2007 issue of *Journal of Strength and Conditioning Research*,[2] found that there was no significant difference in performance or endurance after athletes consumed raisins (a moderate-glycemic food) and a sports gel (a high-glycemic food.)

One word of warning with low-GI foods: Because they tend to be higher in fiber and fat, they will take longer to digest. So you'll want to leave plenty of time between your meal and your run. Also, if your blood sugar is low and you're feeling too tired to run, a low-GI food

CHEW ON THIS

Agave nectar has been touted as a healthy alternative to sugar, because it has a low glycemic index relative to other forms of sugar. But agave nectar has more fructose than the widely demonized high fructose corn syrup (HFCS). Why does that matter? Fructose, unlike other sugars, is metabolized directly by the liver. This can lead to fatty liver deposits, which have been linked to weight gain, insulin resistance, and heart disease risk in animal studies. What's more, as with other forms of sugar, the more you consume, the more you'll crave it. (The fructose in agave nectar should not be confused with the fructose in apples and bananas. While those fruits contain fructose, because of the fiber and other nutrients apples and bananas contain, they're not digested in the same way and don't cause the same kinds of problems as agave nectar and HFCS.)

isn't going to give you the energy surge you need to get out the door. In this case, a high-GI food might be a better choice.

And remember: Just because a food has a low GI number doesn't mean it's healthy. A candy bar, for instance, which no one would list as health food, has a low GI number of 51, in part because its high fat content takes a long time to digest. But that fat is all saturated, which isn't going to help your heart or your long-term health.

During a race or a long endurance event such as a marathon, when you need a quick burst of energy to boost you and prevent the bonk, foods that are higher on the glycemic index are going to be your best bet. They're also ideal right after a hard workout, such as a speed session or a long run, when your muscles need a quick boost of carbs to repair torn muscle fiber and replenish spent glycogen stores. But on an everyday basis, sticking with foods that rank low on the glycemic index is the best way to avoid blood sugar spikes. Because they take longer to digest, they'll help you feel fuller longer.

The GI Index

The GI is not listed on nutrition labels, but you can find a complete list in the international GI database at the University of Sydney in Australia (glycemicindex.com).[3]

Remember that foods are ranked according to 50-gram servings, and a single serving of many foods is more or less than that. Also, the GI only ranks foods with carbs, so it doesn't include meat, fish, or chicken. The following lists, adapted from the International Tables of Glycemic Index and Glycemic Load Values, published in the December 2008 issue of *Diabetes Care*,[4] show where foods rank on the glycemic index.

Low-GI foods (under 55) make great meals and snacks any time of day.

- Chickpeas (10)
- Grapefruit (25)
- Fat-free milk (32)
- Low-fat yogurt (33)
- Pear (38)
- Apple (39)
- Baked beans (40)
- Orange (40)
- Peach (42)
- Dried dates (42)
- Brown rice (50)
- Orange juice (unsweetened) (50)
- Quinoa (53)
- Yam (54)

Medium-GI foods (between 55 and 70) can be consumed in moderation.

- Old-fashioned oats (55)
- Grapes (59)
- Corn on the cob (60)
- Raisin bran (61)
- Banana (62)
- Raisins (64)
- Couscous (65)
- Special K cereal (69)

Reserve high-GI foods (over 70) for midrun energy boosts or postworkout refueling sessions.

- Plain white bagel (72)
- Instant Cream of Wheat (74)
- Gatorade (78)
- Instant oatmeal (78)

- Rice cakes (82)
- White rice (89)
- Corn flakes (93)
- Baked russet potato (111)

THE TAKEAWAY

Make smart swaps. Look at the GI index. See where you can swap low-GI foods for high-GI foods in your regular meals and snacks.

Make room for high GI in your diet. Don't eliminate high-GI foods from your diet; just eat them strategically so you don't feel deprived. And an all-out ban usually leads to a disastrous binge down the road. Pick a high-GI food and reserve it for a preworkout boost or a post-workout treat, when you need fuel fast to bounce back quickly for the next workout. (See Part III for more on when to eat.)

Know the combinations. You can slow down absorption of high-GI foods by combining them with foods with protein, fiber, and fat, which take longer to digest. For instance, you might spread peanut butter on a piece of toast, or top your baked potato with veggie chili.

6

Why Fats Matter

Fats have been another casualty of the dieting mania of the last four decades. The fat-free craze of the 1980s—which ushered in a raft of products for the weight conscious—left us only more overweight decades later.

Like so many other food fads that look to eliminate one group of nutrients altogether, the fat-free craze was a case of a good idea that was taken to an extreme, creating a problem.

It's not that cutting back on fat was such a bad idea. Saturated and trans fats have been linked to higher levels of cholesterol and increased risk of chronic disease, such as heart disease and stroke. And fats do pack a calorie punch, so it's important not to go overboard. (Fat contains 9 calories per gram, compared to carbs and protein, which each have 4 calories per gram.)

But in the rush to extract fat from many popular foods while preserving taste, texture, and shelf life, many manufacturers added in sugars and ingredients such as high fructose corn syrup that kept on fueling overconsumption. Many fat-free yogurts are great examples of this. Check out the sugar counts on the Nutrition Facts and ingredient lists of many popular fat-free yogurts, and you'll see that they violate a lot of the best practices for sugar that we recommended in the previous chapter. So it's no wonder that more than two decades since the tidal wave of fat-free products flooded the supermarket shelves, more than half the population wants to lose weight, and one-third of people report being overweight, according to a Gallup poll.[1]

Fats play an important role in every runner's diet—*especially* if you're trying to lose weight and stay injury-free. Much like carbs, in order to leverage fats to get the results you want, it's important to focus on getting the right kinds of fats and the right amounts.

How Fats Keep You Healthy

Dietary fat helps the body absorb fat-soluble nutrients it needs to log a peak performance, including vitamins D and K, both of which are vital for bone health, and vitamin E, which acts as an antioxidant and helps keep the body from breaking down. Omega-3 fatty acids—the kind found in salmon, walnuts, and ground flaxseed—help fight inflammation and soothe aches and pains. Polyunsaturated fats (PUFAs)—such as the kinds found in avocados, nuts, seeds, and olive oil—have anti-inflammatory properties, so they may help repair the microscopic muscle tears and bone breakdown that happen after a hard workout. And because fats promote the feeling of fullness, they're good for runners who want to shed pounds. They also help prevent blood sugar spikes and crashes, as well as the cycle of craving and overeating that can trip up your training. The right kind of fats—unsaturated—are helpful allies and that's why you shouldn't fear fat. Instead aim for an intake within the recommended range of 25 to 35 percent of your daily calories from fat and make sure the vast majority of fat is from healthy, unsaturated fats.

Still not convinced? There's evidence that a low fat intake is associated with injury risk in female runners. A study in the 2008 *Journal of the International Society of Sports Nutrition* found that injured runners had significantly lower intakes of total fat (63 ± 20 versus 80 ± 50 g/d) and lower percentages of calories sourced from fat (27 ± 5 versus 30 ± 8 percent) compared with noninjured runners. The runners who consumed

CHEW ON THIS

Try to consume as few trans fats as possible. Look for foods that have zero trans fat per serving. But beware: Even if a product claims to be "trans fat–free," it may still have up to 0.5 gram of trans fat per serving. To make sure it's truly free of trans fat, check the ingredient list. If the list includes any partially hydrogenated oil, it has a small amount of trans fat. But if one serving is one cookie and you have more than one, the trans fats can add up.

lower amounts of dietary fat—27 percent rather than 30 percent of daily calories—experienced cases of tendinitis, IT band problems, and more stress fractures than those who consumed the recommended amount.[2]

Know Your (Fat) Type

The *type* of fat you consume makes all the difference in the world. While unsaturated fats can improve your cholesterol and heart health, saturated and trans fats have been found to raise your levels of bad cholesterol (LDL). Trans fats are even worse because they actually lower your good cholesterol levels (HDL). So unfortunately the 11 grams of fat in that honey-glazed doughnut is not going to bestow the same benefits as a tablespoon of avocado and could indeed be hazardous to your health.

As a runner, there's no reason to be afraid of fat but you do need to focus on the kinds of fat you're consuming. Unsaturated fats, such as those from plants, nuts, and seeds—including avocados and olive oil—lower bad cholesterol and help reduce your risk of heart disease.

Unsaturated Fats

These fats lower total cholesterol and LDL cholesterol, and so can help safeguard you against heart disease. You can find these fats in vegetable and nut oils, including almond, avocado, canola, olive, peanut, pecan, and pistachio.

There are two types of unsaturated fats: Monounsaturated fats (sometimes referred to as MUFAs) lower your total cholesterol as well as your LDL cholesterol and have been proven to help reduce belly fat.[3]

The polyunsaturated fats, referred to as PUFAs, have anti-inflammatory properties, so they may help repair muscle tears and bone breakdown after a hard workout. They promote heart health by lowering LDL cholesterol levels.

Some PUFAs—omega-3 and omega-6 fatty acids—are called essential fatty acids. That means the body does not make them, but it needs them for essential functions such as maintaining brain and nerve function. They lower the risk of heart disease and protect against type 2 diabetes, Alzheimer's disease, and age-related brain decline. Because the body does not make them, these fatty acids must be derived from foods.

The American Heart Association recommends that at least 5 to 10 percent of food calories come from omega-6 fatty acids, such as those found in certain oils (corn, soybean, sunflower); nuts and seeds; and certain fish (tilapia).

Two omega-3s—eicosapentaenoic acid (EPA) and docosahexaenoic acid (DHA)—have been found to promote healthy and flexible joints, improve cognition, fight off inflammation, promote a healthy immune system, and bestow a raft of other health benefits. If you're feeling run-down or sore or just want to ensure good health, you might consider adding an omega-3 (fish oil) supplement or consider increasing your intake of fatty fish (which naturally contains omega-3). Fish oil supplements come in various sizes and dosage levels. Look for pills that contain between 1 and 2 grams of EPA and DHA. This means the fish oil might contain more than just 1,000 to 2,000 milligrams total; it's the level of EPA and DHA that's most important. As with other supplements, look for one that's certified by NSF or USP (US Pharmacopeia).

Where the Healthy Fats Are

BEST SOURCES OF HEALTHY FATS FOR RUNNERS

FOOD	FAT CONTENT PER SERVING LISTED	EXTRA NUTRIENTS FOR RUNNERS
Avocado, 1 oz (about ⅕ medium)	5 g	The avocado is an excellent source of monounsaturated fats, which lower levels of bad (LDL) cholesterol and boost heart health. Like most sources of fat, avocado is still dense in calories, so limit your intake to a serving or two a day. Substitute the avocado in place of fats such as butter, cream cheese, or mayonnaise.
Mackerel, salmon, sardines, trout, or tuna, 3 oz cooked	Mackerel = 15 g Salmon = 6 g Sardines = 10 g Trout = 5 g Tuna = 5 g	Fatty fish such as mackerel, salmon, sardines, trout, and tuna contain a healthy dose of omega-3 fatty acids—heart-healthy fats known to fend off heart disease and fight inflammation. The American Heart Association recommends that people eat at least two servings of fatty fish per week. Canned varieties are smart choices; the bones are included, which means you'll boost your calcium intake along with your protein and omega-3 intake.
Olive oil, 1 Tbsp	14 g	Olive oil intake has been linked to reduced risk of stroke and heart disease, as well as improved blood pressure. Olive oil burns more quickly than some other hardier oils. Choose extra-virgin olive oil when you can, since it contains health-boosting antioxidant polyphenols.
Canola oil, 1 Tbsp	14 g	Made from crushed rapeseeds, canola has less saturated fat than any other oil commonly available in the United States. Canola is high in the omega-3 fatty acid ALA, which has been shown to reduce inflammation and improve heart health. Canola is also easy to cook with, given that it has a relatively high smoke point and mild flavor.
Hemp seed oil, 1 Tbsp	14 g	Hard to find and difficult to cook with thanks to a low smoke point, hemp seed oil is an excellent source of omega-3s and polyunsaturated fat. Hemp seed oil should be stored in the fridge. Because of its low smoke point, it is best served cold.
Flaxseed, 1 Tbsp	Flaxseed oil = 13.6 g Ground flaxseeds = 4.3 g	Flaxseed can be an excellent source of heart-healthy fats. Buy ground seeds or cold-pressed oil. (Flaxseeds must be ground to release their nutrients.)
Wheat germ, 2 Tbsp	1.5 g	In addition to providing healthy fats and fiber, wheat germ provides thiamin, an essential B vitamin that converts carbs into usable energy and helps the heart, muscles, and nervous system function properly. It also contains zinc, a nutrient that aids in immune function and healing but is hard to find.

FOOD	FAT CONTENT PER SERVING LISTED	EXTRA NUTRIENTS FOR RUNNERS
Nut butter, 2 Tbsp	Almond = 18 g Cashew = 16 g Peanut = 16 g	Though high in calories, nut butters are a great source of unsaturated fats, fiber, and protein. While peanut butter is certainly the most common variety, almond and cashew butters offer tasty options for those with peanut allergies. Avoid nut butters that contain palm oil or other substitute oils. Look for all-natural nut butters with the fewest ingredients.
Almonds (1 oz or 23 kernels)	14 g	Almonds contain heart-healthy monounsaturated fats, plus they provide vitamin E, an antioxidant that boosts circulation and is hard to find in foods. Studies have shown that eating nuts several times per week lowers levels of LDL cholesterol.
Pistachios (1 oz or 49 kernels)	13 g	Like almonds, pistachios contain vitamin E and heart-healthy fats. They also provide 3 grams of fiber per serving. Pistachios also contain lutein and zeaxanthin, nutrients that are important for eye health. Because you have to work to extract pistachios from the shell, you don't have to worry about getting carried away with snacking.
Walnuts (1 oz or 14 halves)	18.5 g	Walnuts are one of the few plant-based sources of omega-3 fatty acids. While high in calories compared to other nuts, walnuts are still a good choice, as are other nuts; research shows nut eaters are generally thinner and less likely to develop type 2 diabetes; they also have a reduced risk of heart disease compared to non–nut eaters.
Egg (1 whole)	5 g (1.5 g saturated fats)	Whole eggs are a good source of choline (one egg yolk has about 300 micrograms of choline), an important B vitamin that helps regulate the brain, nervous system, and cardiovascular system. Choose omega-3-enhanced eggs to further increase your intake of healthy fats.

Saturated Fats

These fats, often found in animal products such as butter, lard, bacon, beef, lamb, poultry with skin, and full- and low-fat dairy products, can lead to high cholesterol. Some tropical oils, such as palm oil and cocoa butter, also have saturated fats. The American Heart Association recommends limiting intake of saturated fat to no more than 5 to 6 percent of total calories. In other words, if you consume 2,000 calories per day, your intake should be a measly 11 to 13 grams per day, or less than the amount found in 2 tablespoons of butter.

New Questions

For years, health and nutrition experts have urged people to avoid saturated fats as much as possible and recommended that consumers replace them with the heart-healthy mono- and polyunsaturated fats. But recently that advice has come into question.

A review of more than 70 research studies published in the March 2014 issue of *Annals of Internal Medicine*[4] did not find that people who ate higher levels of saturated fat had more heart disease than those who ate less. Nor did it find less disease in those eating higher amounts of unsaturated fat, including monounsaturated fats such as avocados and olive oil or polyunsaturated fats such as soybean and canola oil.

Needless to say, the study stirred a lot of controversy and had many people wondering whether they had the green light to fill their dinner plates with bacon, butter, and sides of sausage.

Not so fast. Decades of research still support the stand that you'll lower your risk of heart disease by replacing saturated fats with heart-healthy fats in nuts, seeds, avocados, fish, plant oils, and vegetable oil soft spreads.

There are no health benefits to saturated fats. But eliminating them from your diet won't make you bulletproof to a heart attack, especially if you replace them with products that have high amounts of sugar. The same holds true for unsaturated fats. Though guacamole has plenty of heart-healthy avocado, if you're using the guac to dress up a bowl of fried chips, you're not doing your body much good.

Trans Fat

While saturated fats have been engulfed in controversy in recent years, on trans fats, sometimes called trans fatty acids, experts universally agree: They're hazardous to your health, and you should eliminate them from your diet or consume as little as possible.

Trans fats became widely used by food makers over the past 30 years because the substance, created when hydrogen is added to liquid vegetable oils, offered a cheap and easy way to extend shelf life and pre-serve flavor in packaged foods.

Decades later, we know how harmful trans fats are to our health. Trans fats increase risk of having a stroke and developing heart disease and type 2 diabetes. Not only do they raise LDL cholesterol like satu-rated fat but they also actually lower HDL cholesterol levels.

In 2006, the FDA began requiring food makers to state how much trans fat packaged foods contained. In 2013, the FDA took it a step fur-ther, determining that intake of trans fats was a "significant public health concern" and they were not "generally recognized as safe," based on evidence that there's no known health benefit. The Institute of Medicine concluded that there's no safe level of consumption.[5]

In response to the backlash, many fast-food chains and food makers have taken trans fats out of their foods and heavily advertised that fact. So when you pick up foods that are free of trans fats, not only will you see a zero in the Nutrition Facts but they're often labeled "trans fat–free."

But what about the foods that don't come in a package? Unless they specifically say "trans fat–free," or free of "partially hydrogenated oils," certain foods are highly likely to contain trans fats. They include:

- Cookies
- Crackers
- Doughnuts
- Muffins
- Pies
- Fried foods
- Cake frosting
- Pancake mixes
- Vegetable shortening
- Spreadable butter and margarine
- Buttered popcorn
- Piecrusts
- Hamburgers
- Beef sausages, hot dogs, and ground beef
- Ready-to-bake cookie dough
- Biscuits
- Ready-to-eat noodles
- Stick margarines

THE TAKEAWAY

Replace bad fats with good fats. If you're taking in saturated or trans fats, swap in healthy forms of unsaturated fats instead.

Make sure you're getting enough healthy fat. Make sure your diet includes at least some healthy fats. At least 15 to 20 percent of your daily calories should come from unsaturated fats. Add avocados to your tuna sandwich, cook with olive oil, or have a 100-calorie pack of nuts as an afternoon snack.

Consider supplementing omega-3 fatty acids. If you have a history of heart disease or you're concerned that you're not consuming enough fatty acids from foods, talk to your doctor about whether you should take supplements.

7

Protein

Scientists have long known that protein builds lean muscle mass and provides a feeling of fullness that can aid in weight loss. A raft of recent studies linking protein-rich diets to weight loss have kept that idea in the spotlight.

In a study in the September 2013 issue of the *FASEB Journal*, people who ate twice the recommended Daily Value for protein while cutting calories and exercising lost more fat and kept more lean muscle than those who stuck with the RDA.[1]

An April 2014 study published in that same journal[2] showed that eating a high-protein breakfast (with 35 grams of protein) curbed appetites later in the day and reduced cravings for high-fat, high-sugar snacks in the evening; it also helped stabilize levels of blood sugar and insulin, thereby reducing risk of diabetes.

Yes, protein is important for weight loss. And as a runner, you need more than what's recommended for sedentary people. That's because as you log miles, you'll need to replace the protein you break down during intense and long workouts in order to build lean muscle tissue.

That said, as with fat and carbs, protein's importance has gotten distorted in the dieting hysteria. Enticed by the link to its proven weight-loss benefits and buoyed by the popularity of low-carb diets, food makers have rushed to add protein to foods such as cereal and granola bars and promote the naturally high protein content of foods such as nuts, beef jerky, and Greek yogurt. There's been a 54 percent increase in the number of new products with a high-protein or vegan claim since 2008, according to Mintel, a London-based research firm.

But not all high-protein products are healthy. Often protein is added to processed and packaged foods along with artificial additives, calories, sugar, fat, and sodium to make the product taste good. So you've got to carefully inspect the Nutrition Facts panel. A 1¼-cup serving of a cereal with added protein, for instance, has 7 grams of protein[3]—more than the 4 grams of protein in the original variety. But it also has about 100 more calories and 16 additional grams of sugar per serving compared to original. Another high-protein candy bar has 20 grams of protein, but it also has other candy-bar-like attributes: 290 calories, 9 grams of fat, and 22 grams of sugar.

It's a confusing time to be a consumer. As is true of the other nutrients, if you want to lose weight, it's important to get the right kinds of protein at the right time and not overdo it.

Why You Need Protein

You need plenty of protein every day. For sure, protein builds muscle, and runners need protein to bounce back quickly from tough workouts. In the 30 minutes following a hard speed session or long run, the body is particularly receptive to protein and carbs to repair muscle tissue and restock glycogen stores. That's why experts recommend that runners have a snack with a 2:1 ratio of carbs to protein in the 30 to 60 minutes following a hard workout such as a long run or a speed session. (To read more, see Chapter 22.)

Protein is also crucial to the regulation and maintenance of the body and plays a role in blood clotting, fluid balance (so you stay hydrated), hormone and enzyme production, and cell repair.

If your protein intake is low, you may start to feel fatigued, lose muscle mass, become run-down, and increase your risk of illness and injury.

Setting Your Daily Protein Target

Protein may be good for you, but it does have calories. So as with carbs and fats, if you consume more protein than you need, it's going to get stored as fat.

Most runners should aim for 0.55 to 0.9 gram of protein per pound of body weight per day to recover from workouts and continue to build fitness. And if you're logging more miles, qualify as a masters athlete, or are incorporating lots of strength training into your routine, you're likely to need more protein. So if you weigh 130 pounds, target 72 to 100 grams per day. A 195-pound runner will need to aim for approximately 107 to 123 grams per day.

It's best to spread that protein intake evenly at meals throughout the day, aiming for an intake of 30 grams at most meals and the remainder at snacks. Protein at each meal and snack will help quiet your appetite, and the 30 grams will make sure that you're eating enough muscle-repairing amino acids at each sitting.

CHEW ON THIS

Look for lean protein on the supermarket shelves. When shopping for packaged foods, pick products that are labeled as "high," "rich in," or "excellent sources of" protein. The FDA requires products that carry those claims to contain 20 percent or more of the recommended Daily Value of protein. When shopping for seafood and meat, look for "lean" on the label. That means the package must contain less than 10 grams of total fat, 4.5 grams or less of saturated fat, and less than 95 milligrams of cholesterol per 100 grams.

Your Best Sources of Protein

Some sources of protein are better than others, and some forms of protein are more readily absorbed by the body. Here are some considerations when choosing your sources of protein.

Go for high quality. Aim to get the protein-rich foods with the most vitamins and minerals and the fewest saturated fats and other ingredients you don't need. Take ground beef. At 23 grams of protein in a 3-ounce serving, a patty made of 90% lean ground beef goes a long way toward helping you boost your daily target for protein intake. But 50 percent of the calories in that serving of ground beef come from artery-clogging saturated or trans fats. So it's best not to make it a part of your everyday diet. Now consider a 3-ounce yellow fin tuna steak, which has 25 grams of protein and just ½ gram of unsaturated fat—with no saturated or trans fats. In this case, tuna is definitely going to be the healthier choice. Just because a food is high in protein doesn't mean it should become a staple of every meal.

Variety matters. Some protein sources are naturally "complete," which means they contain all nine essential amino acids your body needs but can't make on its own. You can find complete proteins in animal-based foods such as steak, fish, pork, and dairy products such as milk, cottage cheese, and yogurts, and some vegetable-based proteins such as soy and quinoa. Other protein sources are considered "incomplete" because they don't contain all nine of the essential amino acids. They must be combined with other foods to provide them. Just take red beans and rice. Eaten alone, the red beans are incomplete. But when eaten in combination with rice, the dish provides the amino acids you need to repair tissue and stave off injury. You don't have to worry about getting these so-called complementary proteins in the same meal. The body can pool nutrients throughout the day. So if one food is low in an essential amino acid, another will make up for it. As long as you accumulate a variety of complete and incomplete proteins throughout the day, you'll be all set.

Pick wholesome sources first. Proteins in some foods are easier for the body to use (or more "bioavailable") than others. In general, you want to try to get a majority of your protein from whole, unprocessed foods, because these foods contain other nutrients your body needs. If you're too pressed for time or don't have access to a refrigerator or cooktop right after a run, you can find high-quality, bioavailable protein in certain protein bars and powders. Because protein is so critical to muscle repair and appetite regulation, it's better to grab a protein shake than to skip it altogether.

When it comes to supplements, choose wisely. The quality of supplemental protein sources, such as protein shakes, is all over the place. If you're reaching for a protein shake, bar, or powdered supplement, here's what to look for.

- **A Nutrition Facts panel:** Packaged foods (such as bars, powders, and shakes), which are highly regulated by the FDA, must have Nutrition Facts panels. Supplements, which are not subject to FDA oversight, carry Supplement Facts panels instead. If a food carries a Nutrition Facts panel, you can rest assured you're getting a high-quality source of protein. Supplements don't need approval from the FDA before they're marketed. The manufacturer of the supplement is responsible for determining that it's safe, and the FDA doesn't test any supplement before it hits store shelves. Also, supplement companies don't have to provide any evidence that their supplement is safe (unless the supplement contains an ingredient that is new to the United States). Plus, once a supplement is on store shelves, it will continue to be sold, even if it's completely ineffective and a waste of money, unless it's proven that the claims of the supplement are false or unsafe. This is not to say that all supplements are unsafe or ineffective; they are not. Many products can be a healthy part of your diet. They're just not subject to the same legal oversight as foods are. Regardless of whether

BEST SOURCES OF PROTEIN FOR RUNNERS

FOOD	PROTEIN CONTENT (G)	EXTRA NUTRIENTS FOR RUNNERS
Chicken breast (3 oz boneless, skinless white meat)	25	Contains selenium, which helps protect muscles from free-radical damage that can occur during running, and niacin, which helps regulate fat burn during a run.
Lean beef (3 oz, 90% lean)	24	Beef boosts iron and zinc to keep your immune system healthy. Choose cuts labeled "loin," "round," or "90% lean."
Pork (3 oz)	22	Pork has iron levels similar to beef but with less fat, plus thiamin, riboflavin, and B vitamins. Look for lean cuts such as tenderloin or loin.
Turkey breast (3 oz boneless, skinless white meat)	22	With only 125 calories, one serving offers more than 50% of your daily niacin and B_6 intake.
Salmon (3 oz)	22	Choose canned for additional calcium. Choose any variety for a healthy dose of vitamin B_{12}.
Tofu, firm (½ cup)	20	A complete vegetarian- and vegan-approved source of protein, a serving of firm tofu set with calcium contains nearly 100% of your daily calcium needs and can help lower cholesterol.
Lentils (1 cup)	18	High in iron, which is vital for transporting oxygen to muscles and organs. Lentils also offer 16 g of fiber per 1-cup serving.
Greek yogurt (5.3 oz)	12–17	This style of yogurt packs more protein, calcium, and vitamin D than traditional yogurts. Aim for low-fat or fat-free varieties.
Chickpeas (1 cup)	12–15	One cup provides 85% of the Daily Value for manganese, which promotes bone health and also helps regulate blood sugar.
Kidney beans (1 cup)	13	Rich in iron, kidney beans are also rich in fiber, providing 11 g per cup.

you choose a protein supplement labeled with a Nutrition Facts panel or a Supplement Facts panel, choose one that has undergone third party testing. Look for products that are certified free of banned substances or certified by NSF, a public health and safety organization.

FOOD	PROTEIN CONTENT (G)	EXTRA NUTRIENTS FOR RUNNERS
Black beans (1 cup)	15	Black beans provide fiber and folate, a B vitamin that plays a key role in heart health and circulation.
Quinoa (1 cup cooked)	8	One of the few vegetarian-friendly foods that provide all the essential amino acids, the building blocks for your body to make more proteins and build muscle. Quinoa also contains fiber and complex carbs.
Milk (1 cup)	8	Contains calcium to build bone health. It's also one of the few dietary sources of vitamin D. To avoid extra calories and saturated fat, opt for low-fat (aim for 1% or less) varieties.
Almonds (¼ cup)	8	Provide vitamin E, an antioxidant that boosts circulation; many runners fall short on it because there are so few good food sources. Almonds also contain heart-healthy MUFAs. Studies have shown that eating nuts several times per week lowers levels of LDL (bad) cholesterol.
Pistachios (1 oz or 49 kernels)	6	Like almonds, pistachios contain vitamin E and heart-healthy fats. They also provide 3 g of fiber per serving. Another benefit of eating pistachios in the shell is that you have to work to eat them, and the left-behind shells provide a reminder of how much you've consumed, so you won't get carried away with snacking.
Egg, whole (1 large)	6	Eggs are rich in protein and choline—a nutrient not found in many foods that is vital for brain health. Choose omega-3-enhanced eggs to increase your intake of healthy fats. And don't lose sleep over the cholesterol found in whole eggs; experts are now recommending folks worry less about cholesterol from foods and more about saturated fat (eggs contain only 1.5 g of saturated fat).
Egg, white (1 large)	3.6	For runners looking to shed pounds but still boost protein intake, one egg white offers a lot of protein for very few calories.

- **Whey, casein, and soy:** Choose a supplement that derives protein from a high-quality source such as whey, casein, or soy, or a blend of all three. Whey, which is derived from milk, is digested quickly and rapidly assists muscle repair and recovery. Casein, also derived from milk, is digested more slowly, so it keeps you feeling full and assists with muscle repair and maintenance for a few hours after you consume it. Soy is digested a little faster than casein but a little slower than whey and is ideal if you're seeking a vegetarian source of protein. If you're a vegetarian, you might also try pea protein. Other types of vegetarian proteins are widely available. In addition to being vegan friendly, pea protein is nearly "complete," so it provides nearly all the amino acids you need for muscle repair. It's also not a risk for anyone with food allergies, generally less expensive than sources of animal protein, and high in arginine, which assists with bloodflow.

Vegetarians

Switching to a plant-based diet can improve your health and won't take anything away from your running. Because vegetarians aren't eating meat—which can be high in saturated fat and cholesterol—and are eating fruits, veggies, and beans that tend to be higher in fiber, minerals, and nutrients, they tend to have lower risks of heart disease, high blood pressure, type 2 diabetes, and cancer.

If you're a vegetarian, you don't necessarily need more protein than meat-eating runners. But you do need to be diligent about meeting your needs. Certain nutrients are harder to get if you're not eating meat—including omega-3 fatty acids, vitamin B_{12}, zinc, and iron.

You can get the protein you need from a variety of soy products, beans, nuts, and whole grains. If you consume a diet rich in these items and other fortified foods you'll be more likely to meet your needs for optimal health as well as performance.

Where to Get It

To boost your protein intake without upping fat, increase the amount of lean proteins you already enjoy: Choose lean ground beef (90 percent lean or higher). Swap in beans for potatoes as a side dish. Use plain, fat-free yogurt as a condiment. And incorporate some protein into breakfast too. When making pancakes or muffins, substitute a scoop of protein powder for a scoop of flour or substitute egg whites for whole eggs to double the protein (four whites equals two whole eggs). And replace your regular yogurt with Greek yogurt, which provides up to four times as much protein as standard varieties.

Protein will help repair torn muscle tissue and keep you feeling fuller longer. For the best sources of lean proteins, and the extra benefits they provide for runners, see the chart on pages 88 to 89.[4]

Amy's Story: **Why Calorie Counting Counts**

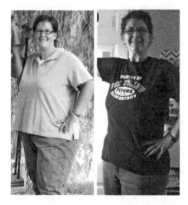

ONCE AMY WHITE hit 300 pounds, there wasn't any question that she wanted to reform her diet and exercise habits; she just wasn't sure how.

"At first I had no clue what to change," says White, 39, a mother of two from American Fork, Utah. "I just knew I shouldn't eat crap food."

She had tried other diets in the past, and while they helped her learn about the value of fruits and vegetables, ultimately it wasn't a sustainable expense, or routine. "Once you quit, if you don't change your lifestyle, it will all come back," says White. "But I couldn't afford it and knew I wanted something permanent."

Money was tight, especially since she recently switched jobs and took a pay cut. After all, if you went to a fast-food restaurant, and everyone ate from the dollar menu, you could feed a family of four for $10 to $15. But she knew her family was paying the price healthwise. "Looking back now, I realize it was a very bad decision on our part," she says. "That's why we'll never go there again."

She downloaded a free calorie-tracking app, which helped her get in the habit of reading food labels. That alone gave her an education in the nutrients she was actually consuming. Realizing how many calories were in her regular fast-food meals made her swear off them altogether.

"Using the app really opened my eyes to calories," she says. "We would go to a fast-food place and I would quickly try to look up the food facts for the place. I realized that I would throw away an entire day's worth of calories plus some by just having a meal."

Her knowledge of calories and nutrients grew, and she got into the habit of turning over packages to read nutrition labels. "After a while I would remember how many calories certain foods were worth," she says, "so it became second nature to look at the back of the packages of food, and I would add it up in my head."

She met with a dietitian, who calculated a daily target for calories, carbs, proteins, and fats. For instance, she realized that with toast for breakfast, a sandwich or two for lunch, and French bread for dinner, she was eating way more carbs than she needed and not enough protein. "It was helpful because I really had to plan everything I ate," she says. "And I could tell the difference when I didn't. I realized that when I stuck to my numbers, I really lost."

Now if the family goes out to eat, she'll have a sandwich wrapped in lettuce instead of bread. Or they'll stop at a place where she can make healthier choices. "We spend a little more money to go to places that serve nicer salads or healthier substitutes," she says.

On a budget of $100 per week for groceries, though, it's tough. "It's hard sometimes, but we make all of our meals at home," she says. Her family stopped eating out as much and made it a once-a-month occasion on payday. "I could feel my body thanking me for this," White says. "It's hard to eat healthy on a limited budget, but I try to buy the least processed stuff every week."

And her family started growing their own food in a garden with tomatoes, bell peppers, lettuce, cucumbers, squash, and zucchini.

White also started running, with the help of a couch-to-5-K app and encouragement from her siblings, who ran her first 5-K at her side. She was hooked and went on to finish nine more 5-Ks, four 10-Ks, and a half-marathon. She has set her sights on a full marathon before her fortieth birthday in March 2016.

Along the way, she lost more than 60 pounds.

It has taken research, trial, and error to figure out how to get the fuel she needs to run hard, without upsetting her stomach. She's researched recipes on the Internet and found inspiring people to connect with online, who are working to achieve similar goals.

"Since I'm still trying to lose weight and get healthier, my body is still changing, and I'm sure I will need to adjust my diet when it comes to running," she says. "But my mind is constantly set on how I can make my runs better, longer, and faster. I don't mind doing research and finding things that work for others, and trying them to see if they work for me too."

THE TAKEAWAY

Figure out how much you need. Aim for 0.55 to 0.9 gram of protein per pound of body weight each day.

Spread your protein intake throughout the day. Protein helps your belly feel full. Make protein a part of each meal and snack to stave off bouts of hunger and cravings.

Focus on natural forms of protein. Avoid products with added protein that have other ingredients you don't need. A good source of protein will have at least 5 to 9.5 grams of protein per serving. A food that is high in protein will have at least 10 grams per serving.

8

What to Drink

If you want to unleash your potential on the road and reach your
weight-loss goals, proper hydration is essential. But that doesn't
mean you have to start buying water bottles in bulk. And it doesn't
mean you have to start lugging around a gallon jug and force-hydrating
yourself. As is true of food, proper hydration involves getting the right
amounts of fluids at the right time.

Why It Matters

Water supports all the major body processes—from regulating your
body temperature to flushing waste products out of your system. All
the organs and cells in the body need water to properly function. Studies have shown that you can't hit the same paces—and by extension,
incinerate the maximum number of calories—when you're dehydrated.[1]
And because the sweating you do through your regular workouts
depletes the water in your system, you need to replenish your stores by
making an effort to hydrate throughout the day and particularly
around your workouts. If you start the next workout dehydrated, it's
going to be slower and feel harder than it needs to be.

Water also has an impact on weight loss. Often the fatigue and drain
that feel like hunger are actually being caused by thirst. So in a fit of
thirst, you may be consuming unneeded calories, when what you really

need is a drink. What's more, when you're dehydrated, you retain water. It's counterintuitive, but it's true. When you're dehydrated, your body works hard to defend and protect you and keep you alive. When it senses that your body is out of balance and not getting the fluids it needs to function best, an antidiuretic hormone is released, which spurs the kidneys (the body's filtering system) to conserve water.[2]

The result? Dehydration could drive up the numbers on the scale—and drive you crazy—unnecessarily. Plus, because water helps you feel fuller, you'll be less likely to overconsume unneeded calories that pack on the pounds.

How Much Do You Need to Drink?

No blanket formula applies for all people all the time. In recent years, hydration experts have concluded that during exercise and the activities of everyday life, simply drinking when you're thirsty will help you stay adequately hydrated.[3]

That said, many people want more concrete directions than simply "drinking to thirst." And because so many people try to satisfy thirst with food instead of water, many nutritionists recommend you drink half your body weight in ounces each day. So if you weigh 160 pounds, aim for 80 ounces per day. If you weigh 130 pounds, aim for 65 ounces. Drink more when it's hotter or if, when you're done with your runs, you have salt streaks on your skin.

Staying hydrated throughout the day is the best way to avoid a last-minute need to pound fluids before a workout, a sloshy or nauseous feeling while you're on the road, and unwanted pit stops on your run. So sip small amounts of water or calorie-free beverages throughout the day.

How do you know if you're well hydrated? When you are, your urine will be the color of pale lemonade or straw. If it's clear, you're drinking too much. If it's the color of apple juice, drink more.

Want a formula for staying hydrated on the run? Do the sweat test. Here's how: Weigh yourself naked before heading out and once again when you return. Keep track of how much fluid you consume during the run and add it to the amount of weight you lose. For every pound of body weight you lose, aim to drink an additional 16 ounces of fluid. Perform the sweat test in different weather conditions, as you'll lose— and need to replenish—a lot more fluid after a hot and humid run than after a perfect, 55-degree day. Record the results and refer to them before you head out on runs.

Which Drinks Hydrate You Best?

Boring as this may sound, water is the best source of hydration for most circumstances. If you can't stand water, reach for a calorie-free form of flavored water or seltzer, or flavor your own with a slice of lemon, orange, cucumber, or mint.

Store shelves are filled with sports drinks that promise to help you go longer, get stronger, run faster, and recover better. Many of them are loaded with calories, sugar, and artificial additives that won't benefit your running and can drag down your weight-loss goals. Whether you need a sports drink is going to depend on the heat and humidity and the length and intensity of your workout.

Many people start pounding the fluorescent-colored sports drinks as soon as they start exercising on a regular basis, because they associate them with being a serious athlete. But the reality is that most of the time, you just don't need them. It's just way too easy to swallow a meal's worth of calories in just a few swigs, and they don't come with the satisfaction and nutrition of a real meal. You don't need a sports drink to hydrate for 8 hours at the office, and unless you're running in Death Valley or an extremely humid environment, you also don't need it after that easy 3-miler.

Special Occasions: When You Need More Than Water

In some cases you need the nutrients that sports drinks provide: carbs for energy and electrolytes such as sodium and potassium, which are critical to nerve and muscle function and are lost through sweat. Here's when to consider adding in something more serious than water.

It's hot and humid outside. When you sweat, you lose electrolytes. Sports drinks will help you restore them and hold on to fluids, so you can keep running strong.

You're running for more than an hour. On any run of an hour or more, you need to refuel on the road with 30 to 60 grams of carbs per hour. If eating on the road gives you GI distress, sports drinks can offer an easy alternative.

You're a salty sweater. If there are white streaks on your skin postrun, it means you've lost quite a bit of sodium and salt through sweating. You have probably also lost other electrolytes such as potassium, magnesium, and even calcium. Sports drinks can help you replenish these electrolytes.

You're doing two runs close together. If you're doing two workouts a day or running in the afternoon, then again the next morning, rehydration is critical to helping you power through the next workout. Complete rehydration involves replacement of both fluid *and* electrolyte losses. After your run, drink 24 ounces of fluid for every pound of weight lost during activity. Water will suffice if you're also eating salty, solid foods. A protein shake with electrolytes will also offer protein, carbs, and fluids for rehydration and recovery. If you can only tolerate fluids and don't have time to digest a protein shake before your next workout, rehydrate by grabbing a sports drink.

Best Sources of Electrolytes

If you want to replenish your electrolytes without the added calories, your best bet is to reach for a low-sugar and low-calorie electrolyte formula. Examine the nutrition label and steer clear of drinks with extra calories, sugars, and artificial sweeteners; look for electrolyte drinks with less than 50 calories per serving. If you want a calorie-free formula, there are many sugar-free drinks and also low-calorie electrolyte tablets, which dissolve quickly in water.

When you've finished a run and are looking for an easy-to-digest and quick drink that rehydrates you and helps your muscles recover, a protein shake can be a great choice. You can make your own, blending some fruit and veggies (try spinach or kale leaves) with a protein powder and 8 to 16 ounces of water or milk plus ice. This combination has water and electrolytes to rehydrate you and protein and carbs to help you recover. If you don't have immediate access to a blender, ready-to-drink protein shakes are the next best choice. (For more, see Chapter 22 on postrun eating.) If you're a salty sweater, add high-sodium vegetables like celery to your shake or try vegetable juice, which is a good source of sodium.

Benefits of Caffeine

One of the most persistent myths is that caffeine causes dehydration. But unless you're consuming large quantities of caffeine, it's okay to drink coffee or caffeinated tea before a workout. (Large quantities—2.7 milli-

CHEW ON THIS

If you're looking to replace electrolytes you lose through sweat, choose a calorie-free sports drink. If it does have calories, choose a drink with less than 50 calories in every 16-ounce serving.

grams of caffeine per pound of body weight per day, or 400 milligrams per day for a 150-pound person—can lead to unwanted side effects for some people. An 8-ounce cup of coffee has about 85 milligrams of caffeine. A 12-ounce cola typically contains about 30 to 40 milligrams of caffeine.) A January 2014 study published in *PLOS ONE* concluded that coffee can hydrate you just as well as water.[4] The study didn't involve runners, but the American College of Sports Medicine says that while caffeine can have a modest diuretic effect in some people, for most people who drink it regularly, it's fine.[5] Studies have shown that caffeine boosts performance; staves off depression;[6] may reduce risk of heart disease[7] and type 2 diabetes;[8] and lessens pain during exercise.[9]

Just avoid making a habit of drinking specialty coffee drinks, or treat them as "sometimes treats." That 16-ounce white chocolate mocha has more than 400 calories—a meal's worth of calories for some—without providing the nutrition or satisfaction of a meal.

And be sure to leave enough time between your java and your run to hit the bathroom. Hot fluids stimulate the bowels (clearing out the system is part of why so many runners rely on prerun coffee), and you don't want to have to make an unwanted stop on the run.

Coconut Water

Coconut water has become the thirst quencher du jour. It's now a permanent fixture in the coolers of convenience stores and natural food stores, alongside traditional sports drinks.

But a closer look at the product offers an enduring lesson on how certain foods and drinks acquire a health halo, when certain nutrition information is swept up in marketing hysteria. It also offers a reminder of why you should look beyond the health claims on food labels before you pick up the habit of consuming any "healthy" processed food on a regular basis.

Coconut water does offer some benefits. It's a natural way to replenish some electrolytes after hard workouts. Unsweetened varieties are free of the sugar, artificial sweeteners, or dyes contained in many conventional sports drinks. And it's high in potassium and magnesium, two nutrients the body needs for general health and good performance and that tend to be lacking in most people's diets. Coconut water has approximately (depending on brand) 600 milligrams of potassium per 8-ounce serving, getting you one step closer to the recommended daily amount of 4,700 milligrams, which few of us meet. Coconut water also offers a handful of other electrolytes like calcium and magnesium. With 60 milligrams of magnesium, an 8-ounce serving provides approximately 15 percent of your daily needs.

However, compared to conventional sports drinks, coconut water is way too low in two of the main ingredients your system needs after a tough workout: sodium, the main electrolyte you lose through sweat, and carbohydrates, which help restock the body's spent energy stores.

So if you're looking for electrolytes to rehydrate during or after a long run, a speed session, or just a tough workout in hot weather, a traditional sports drink is still going to be the best bet to rehydrate and replenish your energy.

While coconut water will replace the small amount of potassium you lose during a workout, it won't replace your sodium losses. But if you're not in the middle of a taxing workout and are simply looking to cut calories and keep your fluids au naturel, coconut water can be a fine choice. Just be sure to reach for unsweetened varieties. For more on how to look beyond food labels, go to Chapter 12.

THE TAKEAWAY

Drink water. Sip calorie-free fluids throughout the day. Aim for half your body weight. So if you weigh 120 pounds, aim for 60 ounces a day. If you weigh 180 pounds, aim for 90 ounces per day.

Watch the color. To determine if you're well hydrated, do the pee test. If you're well hydrated, your urine will be pale yellow, or the color of straw. If you're dehydrated, it will be the color of apple juice. If you're overdoing it, it will be clear.

Reserve sports drinks for special occasions. You only need them for workouts in hot and humid conditions, in which you're losing lots of fluids through sweat or could use the energy boost from carbs that sports drinks contain. Those occasions include speed sessions, runs in hot weather, or runs that last more than an hour. When you're having a sports drink, reach for a low-calorie formula with the least amount of sugar, artificial sweeteners, flavors, and colors, and less than 50 calories per serving.

9

Alcohol

You've likely heard the maxim: Don't drink your calories. But you've probably also noticed that the beer flows freely at finish lines and even aid stations.

Moderate consumption of alcohol can fit into your healthy eating regimen, and it's unlikely to get in the way of your training, as long as you get the timing right. But how much can you drink without seeing the scale go up? And which drink is best nutritionally for the runner looking to lose weight and get faster?

The Benefits of Moderate Consumption

A variety of health benefits have been linked to moderate consumption of alcohol—which the US Dietary Guidelines for Americans defines as no more than one drink a day for women and up to two drinks a day for men. The USDA defines a drink as a 5-ounce glass of wine, 12 ounces of regular beer, or 1.5 ounces of 80-proof distilled spirits.[1]

The benefits include a lower incidence of gallstones, decreased risk of type 2 diabetes, greater bone mineral density, and improved cognitive function in older adults.

For years, those who love red wine cheered the news that a compound it contains—resveratrol—had been shown to contain anti-inflammatory properties, which were thought to reduce the risk of heart disease and even cancer. (Resveratrol can also be found in grapes and dark chocolate with cocoa content of 70 percent or higher.) But a study published in the May 2014 issue of *JAMA Internal Medicine* showed that resveratrol may not be the miracle cure it was once thought to be.[2] Red wine does have catechins, which could help improve "good" HDL cholesterol.

Beer, which also contains ethanol (shown to lower "bad" LDL cholesterol and increase HDL cholesterol), has been associated with a lowered risk of kidney stones in men compared to other alcoholic beverages. Beer is also a source of multiple B vitamins, such as folate, niacin, riboflavin, vitamin B_6, and pantothenic acid, which are involved in hundreds of metabolic reactions that keep the body functioning as a well-oiled machine. While exercise doesn't necessarily increase your need for these nutrients, if you have low intake of vitamins such as B_6,[3] you won't run as well. In general, the more malt in the brew, the more concentrated the level of B vitamins.

What alcohol means to your waistline: If you're watching your weight, it's best to stick with beer or wine, as the calorie counts in mixed drinks and cocktails can vary quite widely, depending on what has been added to them and who is making them.

Treat alcohol like you'd treat a dessert—as a "sometimes treat," advises Karen Ansel, a New York–based registered dietitian and author of *The Calendar Diet*.

CHEW ON THIS

Clearly anyone with a history of alcohol abuse should avoid it completely. Those with other health conditions—such as pregnant women and those at risk of stroke—should also steer clear. Runners with type 1 and type 2 diabetes should be cautious, as alcohol intake can cause hypoglycemia. Alcohol can also wreak havoc with certain medications; if you have a prescription and have questions about whether it's okay to drink, ask your doctor.

If you can limit the number of days you have that drink—and keep the limit to one a day—you can cut down substantially on the amount you drink without feeling totally deprived.

Another thing to note: Once alcohol lowers your inhibitions, you may be more likely to reach for the nachos and dip and less likely to stop when you feel full. "All of a sudden that extra piece of pizza or handful of fries doesn't seem like such a bad idea," says Ansel.

This is especially true if you've been restricting your calories at regular meals. To avoid going off the rails, avoid drinking on an empty stomach. "If you sip your drink while you eat, its alcohol will enter your system more gradually, so you'll make more clear-headed decisions about what and how much to eat," she says.

Delay dehydration by having a glass of water before your first drink and chasing the drink with at least one glass of water afterward. That will also promote a feeling of fullness.

And you may want to stick with beer in a bottle. "It's automatically portion controlled, plus your drink is much larger, so you're less likely to overdo it," Ansel says.

How alcohol affects your training: Downing a few cold ones as you're heading out the door for a run is obviously not a wise move.

While some runners swear that a few beers the night before a race help their performance, the American College of Sports Medicine (ACSM) warns that alcohol affects aerobic power, hurts performance, and impairs the body's ability to regulate its temperature, particularly in cold weather. The ACSM advises runners to skip alcohol for at least 48 hours before a marathon or half-marathon.

Various studies suggest that alcohol intake leads to dehydration (if you've ever suffered from a hangover, you're well acquainted with this), decreases uptake of glucose and amino acids by the muscles, adversely affects the body's energy supply, and impairs metabolic processes during exercise. A study published in the February 2014 issue of *PLOS ONE* showed that drinking alcohol immediately postexercise interferes with the signals that would normally tell your body to adapt and get stronger. So it hampers recovery.[4] So if you want to bounce back quickly from a tough race, it's best to skip that finish-line beer. If you do want to celebrate your finish with a drink, go ahead. Just be sure to rehydrate with water and/or a sports drink first, in addition to eating a healthy recovery meal of protein and carbohydrates.

Bottom line: It's okay to indulge in a drink from time to time. If you want to lose weight, limit it to a "sometimes treat," just as you would with any other food that adds calories—without essential nutrition you need to stay healthy. And if you want to get faster, steer clear of alcohol right before, during, and right after runs.

Allison's Story: Losing the Liquid Calories

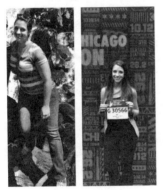

LIKE A LOT OF PEOPLE who lose weight, Allison Taller's game-changing wake-up call came from a photo posted on Facebook.

"I couldn't believe what I was seeing," says Taller, 25, a certification manager from Chicago. "I felt like garbage and I looked like garbage. It was a rude awakening that maybe it was time to start some lifestyle changes."

In college, she would party up to six nights a week, rarely worked out, and ate whatever she wanted, especially late at night. She packed on 20 pounds by graduation.

Once she saw the photos, "I realized I needed to do something for myself," she says. Whenever she felt stress during college, she had been in the habit of reaching for a drink. And that also happened as she became part of the working world. So instead of hitting a bar to relieve a long, stressful day, she started tagging along with her fiancé to the gym after work.

"I started running even though I could barely run half a mile, but the fact that I was outside, moving, and sweating instead of sitting on my butt with a beer was definitely a step in the right direction," she says. "Running became my therapy. My mind truly gets lost when I run, and it's the best escape and reliever of any stresses that may come about in my life."

She downloaded an app and recorded her runs. And it wasn't long before she was hooked. Once a friend suggested a half-marathon, running turned into a hobby and a lifestyle.

"Before I really committed to working out, I felt like I was 'wasting' valuable time by exercising. I wasn't living my life to the fullest or going out and experiencing new things. But once I matched exercise with a feeling of pride and happiness, exercising became my most prideful and essential part of every day," she says.

While running, cutting back on portions, and using smaller plates helped her reform her diet, the biggest change was cutting out alcohol, she says.

One weekend, out of curiosity, she used her app to track how many calories she was drinking and was shocked to see she had consumed more than 2,000 calories just from alcohol in one day.

"That was a huge eye-opener and a true slap of reality," she says. "What was I doing to my body?"

She decided to slowly reduce her drinking, first by looking up the calorie counts and health benefits of different drinks. Once she started reducing her intake, she felt the benefits immediately.

"I still like a glass of wine or craft beer on occasion, but now I know that I like to be coherent and in control instead of letting alcohol drive my life," she says. "If I'm ever stressed nowadays, I find myself grabbing my running shoes instead of a pint of beer."

But it wasn't easy.

"Drinking was such a social habit, and I wasn't really sure what to do in social situations without drinking," she says. After being conditioned in college to drink for fun and in social situations, "you really have to rethink how you interact with people."

Some friends heckled her for easing off the alcohol and told her she wouldn't be as fun. Luckily, her fiancé supported her decision and was proud to see her sticking to her guns.

And she just let her role in social settings evolve to fit her new goals. She volunteered to be the designated driver on big nights out, which gave her, and her friends who were drinking, the assurance that they would all get home safely. "Putting myself in that position allowed me to keep my drinking at bay and also play 'mom' by keeping my friends safe," she says. And when she signed up for a marathon, she wouldn't drink the night before a long run. "It was a bold strategy, but people understood that I was training for a very difficult race and were supportive of that fact."

Because alcohol lowers inhibitions, once she cut back, other calories disappeared too.

"After a night of drinking, what sounds better than pizza or tacos at 2 a.m.?" she says. "And boy, did I feed that want every time."

When she stopped drinking, she noticed she didn't have the same cravings she did before. Plus, since she was tracking her calories and exercise in MyFitnessPal, she learned the difference between true hunger and boredom.

"I realized I felt fresh and healthy when I ate better, and I wanted to keep that feeling going and not undo everything I just did well for the day," she says. She still eats pizza and tacos. "But I know how to eat them within reason now and not to give in at any moment."

After 18 months of running and changes to what she ate and drank, she had lost 30 pounds and reached her goal weight of 133.

"By lowering how much I drank, I became a lot more self-aware in all aspects of my life," she says. "It was probably the best decision I have ever made."

THE TAKEAWAY

Remember moderation. Stick with the Dietary Guidelines and limit drinks to one per day for women and no more than two per day for men.

Get the timing right. Drinking alcohol immediately before a run or race can hamper your performance, and it could lead to injury. But moderate alcohol consumption at other times of day won't hurt and can offer some health benefits.

Wash it down with water. Having water before and after you have alcohol can help promote a feeling of fullness and help prevent the dehydration that alcohol consumption can cause.

10

Sports Foods

Engineered bars, sports drinks, and energy gels are convenient, tasty ways to get the energy boost you need to power through a workout, or recover afterward. But with the explosion of these products in recent years, it can be challenging to figure out which ones actually belong in your diet—especially when you're watching your weight. What's more, many have nutrient profiles that rival common candy bars.

Many people start overdoing it on these bars, shakes, drinks, and gels as soon as they start running regularly. And just like any other excess calories, they can lead to disappointment on your waistline and in your race times. After all, a blueberry-flavored energy bar, which can pack 250 calories, 43 grams of carbs, 21 grams of sugar, and 10 grams of protein, is engineered to get you through a 3-hour-long slow-distance run without hitting the wall. Grabbing one to get

CHEW ON THIS

Sports bars, gels, and drinks can have a place in your diet, even if you're watching your weight. Like so many other foods, it's just a matter of consuming the product that meets your needs for a particular workout without providing calories and additives that you don't need.

through your easy 3-miler or that mind-numbing afternoon staff meeting is definitely overkill.

Choose the Right Bar at the Right Time

If you're going to incorporate engineered foods into your diet, become a label detective. Make sure you know you're getting the amount of calories, fat, carbs, fiber, and sugar you need for a specific workout. And be sure to read "serving size" carefully. Many bars packaged as single servings actually contain two.

You're going to need to experiment with different products and flavors to figure out what gives you a boost without upsetting your stomach. Here's what to look for in different situations.

Prerun snack: Choose products high in the muscle-fueling carbs you need to energize your workout but low in the fat and fiber that could lead to GI distress on the road. For a run of 60 minutes or less at an easy effort, limit it to 200 calories or less, with less than 10 grams of fat, 10 grams of protein, and 7 grams of fiber.

Midrun refueling: Choose products high in the carbs you need to sustain energy over a long period of time, and again, low in fat and fiber that could upset your stomach. If you're going to be on a run for 1, 2, or 3 hours, you want to aim for a product that provides 30 to 60 grams of carbs per hour you're on the road.

Postrun refueling: In the 30 to 60 minutes right after a long run or a tough speed session, your body is extra primed to absorb carbs and protein to rebuild muscle tissue so you can bounce back strong. After a speed session or a long run, a sports bar with a 2:1 ratio of carbs to protein is ideal to help you bounce back strong. For more, see Chapter 22.

Meal replacement: At mealtime it's best to have, well, a meal. But if you're in a rush and need something quick to keep your appetite from kicking into overdrive, it's okay to reach for an engineered bar. Just make sure the bar doesn't contain more calories than you'd have in a regular meal. Look at the serving size; some bars have more than one serving in a bar, and look for an option that contains a balance of carb, protein, fat, and fiber. The best bar will contain at least 10 grams of protein and 5-plus grams of fiber because that's what you'd be consuming if you chose whole foods instead.

Strength-training session: A strength-training workout requires hard work. So fueling up beforehand is critical. You want to feel energized and strong heading into the workout; if you feel weak or famished, you might be tempted to skip reps or use momentum instead of muscle to go through the motions. While some strength athletes consume protein during workouts to maximize the impact, it's unnecessary for most runners. If you simply want to get stronger, tone up, trim your waistline, and prevent injuries, you don't need to fuel up mid-workout. During your strength workout, sip on water to prevent dehydration. If you start feeling dehydrated and develop muscle cramps, add a low-calorie or calorie-free electrolyte drink. Just like you would after a tough run, once you've finished your strength session, have a recovery meal or shake within 30 to 60 minutes of completing the workout. Aim for an intake of 15 to 25 grams of protein with two to four times as much carbohydrate.

Even when you're looking for a convenient prerun or preworkout snack, plenty of good, portable whole-food alternatives will fuel you just as well and don't require spending valuable time trying to decode the Nutrition Facts label. With whole foods—such as apples, oranges, and bananas—you're getting vitamins and minerals you need along with your energy boost, without having to worry about additives that you don't need or that might upset your stomach. You can see more prerun snacks on page 167.

Read the Ingredients

Look at the Nutrition Facts label on these products, and you're likely to see a lot of ingredients you can't pronounce, much less make an educated decision about ingesting. Here's a guide, compiled by *Runner's World* contributor Kelly Bastone.[1]

Maltodextrin: This lab-formulated carbohydrate is more quickly absorbed than other carbohydrates, so it delivers a fast hit of fuel. It's also easier on the stomach than the concentrated glucose found in some sports drinks. Because maltodextrin is relatively tasteless, it's a useful choice if overly sweet gels and chews don't sit well with you.

Protein (whey and soy) isolates: Whey and soy proteins are first extracted from a food and then added to bars to boost protein content. Hydrolyzed proteins undergo further processing that removes vitamins but makes the protein more digestible.

Glucose syrup: It's another term for corn syrup. It's used because it bonds easily with dry or solid ingredients. Its short, simple sugar chains are rapidly absorbed, so it offers instant fuel that's ideal for prerun energy.

Sugar alcohols: Sugar alcohols, such as sorbitol, xylitol, maltitol, mannitol, and isomalt, are reduced-calorie sweeteners often found in sugar-free and no-sugar-added products such as ice cream, candy, cookies, and chewing gum. Sugar alcohols provide fewer calories than sugar and have less of an effect on blood glucose (blood sugar) than other carbohydrates. While they tend to have fewer calories than their sugar-filled counterparts, it's important not to go overboard. Consuming sugar alcohols can lead to GI distress, and they can have a laxative effect.[2]

Brown rice syrup: This sweetener is a bit higher in nutrients and is slower-burning than corn syrup. But organic versions can contain traces of arsenic, which is naturally present in the soil. Its health threats haven't been confirmed, but some companies may stop using it.

THE TAKEAWAY

Shop around. Try different brands and flavors to figure out which products give you a boost without upsetting your stomach.

Use 'em, don't abuse 'em. Think about the occasions when you have engineered sports foods such as energy or protein bars. Are you using them to fuel up your workouts and recover afterward? Or are you using them as snacks and pick-me-ups when you don't really need them?

Find whole-food alternatives to engineered foods. By sticking with wholesome sources of energy, you get more of the vitamins and minerals you do need and less of the additives and calories you don't.

11

Artificial Sweeteners

For anyone watching their weight, diet sodas, low-calorie foods, and sugar-free treats seem like gifts from the gods. They seemingly give you the green light to enjoy your favorite sweets without getting weighed down by the guilt or the calories that their full-calorie counterparts contain.

But if you're trying to lose weight and get faster, are foods made with calorie-free sweeteners a wise choice? While zero-calorie versions of foods can make it easier to meet daily calorie goals, new questions have emerged about whether, over the long term, they help—or actually hinder—weight-loss efforts.

Safety Concerns

After decades of research, US health authorities have deemed that all the popular sweeteners on the market—from aspartame to Splenda—are safe. Studies in the early 1970s linked saccharin to bladder cancer in lab animals, and for years saccharin carried a warning label saying so. But by 2000, after subsequent research, the FDA removed the warning label, having concluded that there was enough evidence proving its safety in humans.[1]

Artificial Sweeteners: Do They Help or Hurt Weight Loss?

So artificial sweeteners help you meet your daily calorie targets. But are they the best bet for long-term weight loss?

Sugar-free doesn't always mean healthful, says registered dietitian Jenna A. Bell, PhD, director of food and wellness at Pollock Communications, a New York–based consulting firm. If you're limiting your calorie intake but really, really want a cookie or some hot chocolate, the sugar-free version is going to save you calories. But that doesn't mean it's good for you. Most of the time, baked goods, ice cream treats, and candies that are sugar-free don't offer any nutritional benefits. And they still have calories. So if you go overboard, you're still going to see the results on the scale.

And there's plenty of evidence that consumers *do* tend to go overboard when eating diet food. A study published in the November 2006 issue of the *Journal of Marketing Research* found that people ate up to 50 percent more of food that was deemed "low fat."[2]

Diet Drinks

Health authorities such as the Academy of Nutrition and Dietetics have concluded that diet drinks are associated with weight loss and don't affect appetite for food. And certainly, if you want to shed a lot of pounds and you drink a lot of soda, swapping your full-calorie variety for a diet version will make an impact. Consider this: If you drink three regular soft drinks per day, you're consuming in excess of 400 calories, which adds up to about 3.5 pounds over the course of a month. If you simply switched to diet soft drinks and made no other changes, you'd be likely to lose that 3.5 pounds instead of gaining it.

That said, research has emerged in recent years that actually links carbonated diet drinks to higher risks of belly fat, weight gain, and chronic diseases.

A study published in the June 2010 issue of the *Yale Journal of Biology and Medicine* concluded that "artificial sweeteners, precisely because they are sweet, encourage sugar craving and sugar dependence."[3] A study published in the April 2015 issue of the *Journal of the American Geriatric Society*[4] found that diet soft drink users had 70 percent bigger waist sizes than nonusers. Those who drank two or more diet sodas a day had waists that were five times bigger than those of nonusers. What's more, we hear plenty of anecdotes from runners who report that giving up diet drinks gave their weight-loss efforts and running a lift.

"I felt sluggish when I would drink soda, but I was hooked on it," says Amy White, a mother of two from Utah who lost 102 pounds. "It wasn't until I really stopped drinking it altogether that I felt I could go faster, longer, and harder. I have the occasional soda, and I always regret it afterward because I can feel it messing with my body."

Ditching Diet Soda

By Ted Spiker

Recently a friend came to a group workout with a see-through water bottle minus the water. The liquid looked dark like potting soil, not rainbowy like a sports drink, so I asked if she was going with iced coffee to power her through the next hour.

"No," she said. "Diet Coke."

I wondered aloud how diet soda could serve as a thirst quencher for a strenuous stretch of sweat. She just shrugged and said that's what she always drinks during training.

I got it.

Though exercise was the one time I didn't have a Diet Coke by my side, I spent the better part of two decades addicted to the beverage. When I met my now-wife, that's what she drank. Never one to drink much soda until that point, I tried it with a meal. And oh-my-wow, was it good with a burger. And with a sandwich. And with breakfast. And after a run.

I drank it again and again until it morphed from new habit to full-on addiction. My diet soda (I gladly rotated in Diet Dr Pepper, Diet Cherry Coke, and diet cream soda) became such a part of my day that I had to measure my intake in gallons, not glasses. I'd have it in the morning at my desk, make several trips to a fountain for lunch, have more to get through the afternoon, then refill and refill and refill at dinner and through the night.

I drank so much diet soda, I think my blood was carbonated.

As someone who has struggled with my weight my entire life, it made sense. Why not drink something that tastes sweet but has zero calories? Surely that was better than regular soda or juice or cookie-dough milkshakes.

But one day in the summer of 2011—during a time when the scale decided to frustrate me with some serious back talk—I decided to stop.

Just quit it all.

Deep down, I knew that diet soda wasn't to blame for my creeping weight levels (though one of my impetuses surely came from the mounting evidence that diet drinks are linked to weight gain and other health issues, seemingly because they mess with hormone levels that influence hunger). It wasn't the no-calorie drink that made me gain weight, but rather the megacalorie everything else. Still, I wanted to do something, and I wanted to show that I could control the one thing I couldn't.

So on a July day in 2011, I just stopped. I started drinking more water and more coffee.

And I went from being a Diet Coke addict to a Diet Coke ex.

I remember wanting some on the first day or two after my stoppage, but the newness of the experiment gave me the initial will to make it through those days. After that, nothing. No desire. No slip-ups (minus a rogue sip I took when I messed up cups with my wife).

I realized that my habit wasn't as much about the taste as it was about having something in my hand, at my desk, something to occupy my mouth so it didn't detour to the Doritos.

Two years after I stopped, I started training for an Ironman at the urging of my friend. We spent a lot of time talking about nutrition, and one of the staples of Ironman training, he told me, was regular Coke. When you're spending that much time on the bike or running, that little jolt of immediately available sugar and caffeine would help get you through, he said.

"You don't understand," I said. "I gave up soda. I don't drink it anymore."

Eventually he convinced me that this situation was different, that regular soda wasn't diet (and that's what my addiction was to), and that the needs of my body in these training moments superseded my artificial achievement of going cold turkey on cold soda.

I eventually caved to the siren of sugar. During and after long rides in the 90-degree Florida August, I replenished with a Coke.

It. Was. Bleeping. Fabulous.

Throughout the next months, I drank regular soda in conjunction with training, not at meals, and I loved it.

After the race was all over, I wondered if I'd slip back—to a new addiction or maybe back to my old one.

Now, some years later, I haven't.

I haven't really missed it either. Occasionally—like after a long run or if I see my wife's 44-ouncer with crushed ice on the counter—I'll get a ping in my tongue that says, "Sure looks good." But I haven't given in to the fleeting temptations (though writing about it now makes one sure sound good).

I don't know if my giving up diet soda has made any difference internally. Maybe I'm healthier. I know I'm lighter than I was that day in 2011 (though that's due to a variety of factors). I do feel cleaner.

More important, it made me realize that I could face a weakness— and do something about it.

Ted Spiker is the author of Runner's World *Big Guy blog, author of* Down Size, *and 2013 last-hour Ironman Florida finisher.*

THE TAKEAWAY

Make your calories count. Remember, foods should provide nutrients that keep your body in its best shape. Before indulging in foods sweetened with sugar substitutes, ask how nutritious the food is. Low-calorie does not necessarily translate to "good for you."

A "diet" label isn't license to go overboard. It's easy to overdo it on foods that are labeled as low in fat. Remember: Extra calories are extra calories, even when they come from diet foods.

When in doubt, cut it out. If you're wondering whether diet foods are keeping you from feeling your best, cut them out for a week and see how you feel. You may be surprised by the results.

12

Decoding Food Labels

O ne of the most powerful tools you can use to reach your feel-great weight and your dream time on the finish line is hidden in plain sight: It's on the nutrition label of your favorite packaged foods.

Studies have shown that people who read food labels are more likely to lose weight than those who don't.[1] And many dieters and runners find that reading food labels is both surprising and humbling. They're often shocked to find out how many calories a small snack they might not have thought about actually contains, or to realize that they're consuming half a day's worth of calories in the car on the way home from work. There's plenty of evidence that when left to our own devices, we vastly underestimate calorie counts.[2]

But deciphering what those labels mean—and determining which foods are going to help you reach your goals—isn't always easy. From *gluten-free* to *no high fructose corn syrup* to *non-GMO* there's been a barrage of

CHEW ON THIS

Don't get derailed by a health halo. While terms such as *gluten-free* may be important for people with celiac disease, and *non-GMO* may be important for those worried about genetically modified ingredients, those terms do not necessarily mean the foods are going to help you achieve your weight-loss goals. Read the food label with your personal weight-loss priorities in mind.

so-called health halos, some of which have no legal definition; many of these claims can lead you to overestimate the nutritiousness of a food.

Here are some tips on how to scrutinize labels so you find the products that will help you meet your goals. To find out what terms such as *low fat* mean, see page 270. For a 12-step quick guide to reading a food label, turn to page 121.

Hold yourself to high standards. The FDA has established standard definitions for certain claims, but not others. For instance, foods labeled "low calorie" cannot have more than 40 calories per serving. Claims such as "low carb," "low sugar," and "natural" sound nutritious but aren't required to meet any FDA standard. You can find a quick guide to FDA-approved definitions of some of the most common claims at eatright.org.[3]

Watch your portions. Even if a health claim is legitimate, it's not a license to go overboard. Excess calories can lead to weight gain—even if they come from healthy foods. A study in the November 2006 issue of the *Journal of Marketing Research* found that people who were given a food labeled "low fat" ate 50 percent more than those who ate the regular version.[4] Some foods that look like a single serving are actually two servings, or even more. So read the "serving size" before you eat.

Prioritize. What to look for depends a lot on your unique health concerns. If you have high blood pressure, you may want to look for products labeled "salt- or sodium-free" that have less than 5 milligrams of sodium per serving. Or look for the American Heart Association's "Heart Check" seal of approval,* which shows that a product meets certain nutrition requirements.

Don't forget the ingredients. Ingredients are listed in descending order from highest percentage to lowest. So the ingredients listed first are the ones included in the largest amounts. If the ingredient is toward the end of the list, the product contains a small amount. So if you're trying

---

* To learn more, check out the AHA's page on heart-smart shopping at heart.org
/HEARTORG/GettingHealthy/NutritionCenter/HeartSmartShopping/Heart-Smart
-Shopping_UCM_001179_SubHomePage.jsp.

to steer clear of sugar, for instance, make sure added sugars are not among the first few items on the ingredient list. And know that sugar goes by a lot of other names. If a product says that there's "no sugar added," it contains no table sugar or any other sugar-containing ingredient but the product may include other naturally occurring sugars such as fructose and lactose. For example, yogurt may have no sugar added, but the lactose in the milk naturally provides low amounts of sugar. Foods labeled "no high fructose corn syrup" may sound healthier, but if they're higher in other sugars such as evaporated cane juice, agave syrup, brown rice syrup, or even apple or grape juice concentrate, they're no healthier.

Gluten-free does not necessarily mean good. The term *gluten-free* is critical for anyone with celiac disease—a digestive condition in which gluten damages the small intestine and causes other health problems. But lots of people buy gluten-free foods on the assumption that they're automatically healthier. That's just not necessarily true. Indeed, scores of potato chips, cookies, and candy bars sport the "gluten-free" label. And many gluten-free foods have refined carbs and added fats. So be sure to check out the other vital stats on the package to make sure the calories, fats, sugars, and other ingredients are going to help you achieve your weight-loss goals. See Chapter 1 for more on carbs.

Eco-friendly does not always mean diet-friendly. The "certified organic" label means the food is grown without pesticides, antibiotics, or growth hormones. But now that many cookies, candies, and other not-so-diet-friendly items are organic, you should still closely examine the Nutrition Facts panel and ingredients. Likewise, foods labeled "non-GMO" (containing no genetically modified organisms), this is meant to distinguish them from foods that have been genetically altered to increase resistance to damage from things such as pests and disease.* While labels such as "organic" and "non-GMO" may be good

---

* More than 22,000 products now bear a "Non-GMO Project Verified" seal from the non-profit group based in Bellingham, Washington. To learn more, visit nongmoproject.org /find-non-gmo/search-participating-products.

for the farmer or the environment, if you're concerned about your weight, they're not the most important variable.

For a full chart of what different labels mean, go to page 270 in the back of the book.

When you're examining the Nutrition Facts panel and ingredient list on your favorite foods, here's your 12-step guide to what you should look for to lose weight and get faster.

1. **Serving size:** Many serving sizes are much smaller than what people are accustomed to eating. To stay on track, you may want to break out your measuring cups, spoons, and kitchen scale.

2. **Number of servings:** Some foods that look like a single serving are actually two servings or even more.

3. **Calories per serving:** Assess this in terms of your daily calorie targets. (See Chapter 16 for more on how to set realistic calorie targets to lose weight and get faster.) If your daily calorie target is 1,600 and that smoothie has 600 calories, you'll need to figure out how to cut back in other places.

4. **Trans fats per serving:** Avoid them altogether. In November 2013, the FDA took them out of the "generally recognized as safe" category. The Institute of Medicine has concluded that trans fat provides no known health benefit and that there's no safe level of consumption of artificial trans fat.[5]

5. **Saturated fat per serving:** Eating foods that contain saturated fats raises the level of cholesterol in your blood. High levels of saturated fat increase your risk of heart disease and stroke. So keep your intake as low as possible. The American Heart Association recommends no more than 5 to 6 percent of your daily calories from saturated fat. So if you aim for 1,600 calories a day, you shouldn't consume more than 9 to 11 grams of saturated fat per day.

6. **Sugar per serving:** Aim as low as possible, no more than 10 grams of sugar per serving. To keep your energy levels stable, try to consume this at even intervals throughout the day. If you're craving an item with more sugar, have it right before a workout, when your body can use it for energy, or within 30 minutes of finishing a tough workout, when your body needs carbs to restock your glycogen stores so you can bounce back for your next workout. (Adding protein to that sugary snack will speed up this process. To read more, turn to Part III on when to eat.) And if you're eating raw fruit or a dairy product, don't stress about sugars.*

7. **Protein per serving:** Aim for as high as possible, while still maintaining your calorie target for your meal or snack. Protein helps repair and rebuild torn muscle tissue so you can bounce back strong for your next workout. And it promotes a feeling of fullness, so you won't feel hungry. That's why it's important to spread protein intake evenly throughout the day. But watch out for some seemingly healthy, "high-protein" foods. Some items, such as high-protein bars, may have a meal's worth of protein, but they also have a meal's worth of calories, at 300 to 400 calories per bar. There are better choices out there.

8. **Fiber per serving:** Like protein, fiber makes you feel full. It also keeps your GI tract healthy and, because it can reduce your cholesterol levels, fiber promotes heart health. Men should aim for 38 grams of fiber per day and women should

---

* The American Heart Association says women should limit added sugars to 100 calories or 25 grams per day; men should have no more than 150 calories or 27.5 grams per day. But on today's nutrition label, it's nearly impossible to determine how much of the sugar in a product comes from unhealthy additives and how much sugar occurs naturally, such as fructose and lactose, and so is not as unhealthy. To make things easy, try to keep it under 10 grams per serving and don't stress out about amounts of sugar in raw fruits or milk.

target 25 grams of fiber per day. So aim as high as possible with fiber. But to avoid GI distress on the run, your pre-workout snack or meal should have less than 7 grams of fiber per serving.

9. **Vitamins and minerals:** The best foods are nutrient dense, which means that in addition to having a good blend of carbs, fats, and protein, they contain a smattering of vitamins and minerals you need to stay healthy, such as calcium, vitamin C, iron, and B vitamins. Look at the "recommended daily allowance" column to see how high the product is in these essentials.

10. **Ingredient list:** Remember, ingredients are listed in descending order, according to weight. So the ingredients near the front of the list are in a higher proportion than the ingredients near the back. If you see sugar in any of its other forms (see Chapter 4 for more details) listed in the first three ingredients, choose another food. Also beware that even if it's not in the first three ingredients, if you see lots of other forms of sugar throughout the list, it can add up.

11. **Sodium:** Aim for less than 200 milligrams per serving most of the time. Most adults should reduce intake to no more than 2,300 milligrams per day (and those at risk of heart disease need even less). Runners can get away with a higher intake of sodium (since sodium is lost via sweat) but you'll still want to watch for sodium in canned goods, processed foods, and sauces, and use fresh options whenever you can.

12. **Cholesterol:** Because cholesterol has been linked to a higher risk of heart disease, keep intake as low as possible. Focus on reducing intake of saturated fat and trans fat, as they drive up levels of LDL or "bad" cholesterol in the blood.

THE TAKEAWAY

Read food labels for 1 week. Use the quick guide on page 270.

Remember your portions. Some of the healthiest foods can still derail your diet if you eat multiple servings in one sitting. Check serving sizes. Use measuring cups and spoons to see what an actual portion looks like on your plate.

Don't get tricked by packaging claims. Some claims have no legal definition, and others (such as "organic" or "natural") may sound healthy, but that doesn't mean the food item behind the label is the best choice for you.

CHAPTER

13

Vitamins and Supplements

Vitamins and minerals play many important roles in your health. They're critical in helping your body turn food into energy, keeping bones strong, boosting your immunity, and repairing and rebuilding muscle.

And because exercise taxes many of the basic body functions and systems where vitamins and minerals play a key role, health authorities such as the American College of Sports Medicine and the Academy of Nutrition and Dietetics have concluded that runners may need to make an extra effort to get those vitamins and minerals.[1]

It's always best to get vitamins and minerals from foods rather than supplements. Your body absorbs them better. Unless you're eating an unbalanced diet that consists of only one or two food items all the time, you don't run the risk of building up certain nutrients to toxic levels. And if you load up on fresh vitamin- and mineral-rich fruits and vegetables, you get other important nutrients such as phytochemicals and fiber that you miss out on if you just pop pills.

But when you simply can't consume enough foods to meet your nutrient needs—whether it's because you're cutting back your intake, have food allergies, or just don't like certain foods—it's a good idea to take a supplement.

While no vitamin or mineral is magically going to help you lose weight, certain deficiencies can prevent you from meeting your weight-loss and racing goals. If you're not getting enough vitamin D or calcium, for instance, you could put yourself at risk of stress fractures. And that can sideline you for months from running. If you're low in B_{12} or you don't absorb it properly, you might feel chronically fatigued and unable to give your all to workouts and burn as many calories.

How do you know if you have a nutrient deficiency? You won't know until you run into a problem (say you start to get injured frequently or feel chronically run-down), see a doctor, and get a blood test. So think of taking a multivitamin as having insurance; even if you don't need coverage for all the nutrients and minerals all the time, they'll be in good supply when you do need them.

Many sports foods are fortified with essential nutrients. So if you regularly eat engineered foods such as energy bars or protein shakes, you're likely getting the essential nutrients you need.

- **Read the labels:** When you're shopping, certain seals of approval on the product labels can give you confidence that the pills you're buying actually provide the nutrients and minerals they claim to contain.

- **USP:** This is the logo of the US Pharmacopeia. Products that carry this seal have voluntarily submitted to a third-party verification program and met stringent testing and auditing criteria set by a third party.

- **NSF:** This is another third party that tests ingredients and products to make sure they're safe, they follow good manufacturing processes, and what's on the label is in the bottle.

The nutrients runners need most: If you've been cutting calories, increasing mileage, following a strict diet, doing a detox, or eliminating food groups, you may be at risk of nutrient deficiencies, and a supplement might be right for you. See the chart beginning on the opposite page for some of the nutrients runners need most.

BEST NUTRIENTS FOR RUNNERS

	WHY RUNNERS NEED IT	BEST SOURCES FROM FOOD	DAILY DOSAGE
Vitamin D	The body needs vitamin D to absorb calcium and regulate phosphorus to keep your bones healthy. If you train mostly indoors or live in a place with limited sunshine, you're at risk of vitamin D deficiency.	Dairy is the main source of vitamin D; it can be hard to find in other foods. Look for products fortified with vitamin D, such as breads, orange juice, and margarine, as well as mushrooms grown under UV lights.	Athletes with insufficient intake or who live in northern states or Canada may benefit from a vitamin D supplement. Look for one that meets the recommended Daily Value of 600 IU/day.
Calcium	Runners who restrict calories—especially female runners—tend to have low intakes of this bone-building and bone-repairing nutrient. Calcium plays a role in many basic body functions, including muscle contraction and blood clotting. If your diet is low in calcium, you'll likely be draining it from your bones. If you don't get enough calcium and vitamin D, you increase the risk of low bone-mineral density and stress fractures.	Dairy products can help you meet most of your calcium needs. It can also be found in products that are made with milk (such as crackers and breads), canned salmon, tofu set with calcium carbonate, and fortified orange juice. Leafy greens are a source of calcium, but it is not as well absorbed by the body as the calcium in other products.	Most adults need 1,000 to 1,200 mg per day. But if you're at risk of osteoporosis, struggling with disordered eating, severely restricting calories, or have amenorrhea, you need more—up to 1,500 mg of calcium per day. Your body can only absorb 500 mg of calcium at a time, so break your intake into two to three smaller doses.
B vitamins: thiamin, riboflavin, niacin, B_6, pantothenic acid, biotin, folate, and B_{12}	All B vitamins are essential for energy metabolism. Thiamin, riboflavin, niacin, B_6, pantothenic acid, and biotin aid in energy production during exercise, while folate and B_{12} are required for red blood cell production, protein synthesis, and tissue repair. Female athletes, especially vegetarians or those with disordered eating patterns, are often low in riboflavin, pyridoxine, folate, and B_{12}.	Enriched and whole grains are a potent source of many B vitamins. Other sources include meat, nuts, dairy, and green vegetables.	Some data suggest that exercise may increase the need for B vitamins by as much as twice the current recommended amount. Other experts suggest that as long as you're eating enough, you're fine. But if you're limiting calories to lose weight, you may want to consider adding a supplement. Look for one that provides 100% of your daily needs. If a supplement isn't for you, focus on consuming foods rich in B vitamins.

(continued)

BEST NUTRIENTS FOR RUNNERS (CONT.)

	WHY RUNNERS NEED IT	BEST SOURCES FROM FOOD	DAILY DOSAGE
Iron	For runners, iron plays a vital role in forming oxygen-carrying proteins, hemoglobin, and myoglobin. Without enough iron, you're likely to fatigue easily and feel winded before you finish your run. Low levels of iron can impair muscle function and limit your exercise capacity. Iron is one of the most prevalent deficiencies in athletes, especially female athletes. A number of factors can lead to iron deficiencies, including vegetarian diets, inflammation, heavy sweating, menstrual periods, and foot strike hemolysis.	It's easiest for the body to absorb heme iron—the kind that comes from animal products, such as beef, pork, poultry, and liver. If you don't eat meat, nonheme iron sources such as black beans, kidney beans, fortified grains, and breakfast cereals are good options. For best absorption pair iron-rich foods with foods that are high in vitamin C, like citrus fruits, leafy greens, and red peppers.	For nonrunners, the Institute of Medicine recommends that women get 18 mg of iron per day; the RDA for men is 8 mg of iron per day.[2] Runners should aim for 1.3 to 1.7 times those levels, as they naturally lose iron during exercise. Vegetarians should also aim for that intake because vegetarian (nonheme) sources of iron are not as well absorbed as animal (heme) sources.
Zinc	Zinc plays a role in immune function, hemoglobin production, energy production, and building and repair of muscle tissue.	Find zinc in red meat, dark-meat poultry, raw oysters, whole grains, wheat germ, and enriched grains and cereals.	Men need 11 mg of zinc per day; women need 8 mg per day, but many individuals in the US do not consume the recommended amount of zinc. Zinc is not always readily absorbed, as other nutrients can interfere with bioavailability. For example, if you're taking a nonheme iron supplement, you'll want to pay close attention to your zinc intake, as nonheme iron can inhibit zinc absorption. Heme iron (the kind in red meat) doesn't have the same effect. Your best bet is to keep your diet high in zinc through daily consumption of some of the foods listed in the column on the left.

	WHY RUNNERS NEED IT	BEST SOURCES FROM FOOD	DAILY DOSAGE
Magnesium	Magnesium is a key mineral for strong bones; it helps to regulate calcium balance and vitamin D balance. Magnesium is also critical to nervous system functions, blood sugar control, protein synthesis, and blood pressure regulation. Marginal magnesium deficiency can actually impair performance as well as amplify the negative effects of strenuous exercise.	Magnesium is found in leafy green veggies such as spinach as well as many whole grains, seeds, and nuts. Seafood, beans, and dairy products also contain some magnesium. Refined and processed foods are generally low in this nutrient.	Men ages 19 to 30 should take 400 mg per day; men over 30 should aim for 420 mg per day. Women ages 19 to 30 should aim for 310 mg per day; after the age of 30 women should aim for 320 mg per day.

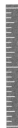

CHEW ON THIS

Because many vitamins can cause GI distress, you might want to take your vitamins before bed, when you have plenty of food in your stomach. If you've been prescribed a supplement by a doctor, find out if a certain time of day is best to take it and whether it should be consumed with food or on an empty stomach.

Single supplements or multivitamin? Is it better to take a multivitamin or a single supplement such as D_3 or omega-3? In general, a multivitamin should meet your needs if you eat a varied diet and the supplement provides close to 100 percent of the recommended daily allowance (RDA) of nutrients. Various nutrients—such as vitamin D, calcium, and iron—can be difficult to get in sufficient amounts in a multivitamin and may warrant a supplement if you have been diagnosed with a deficiency. But if you have not, just stick with a multivitamin. Single-nutrient supplements tend to supply much more than 100 percent of your needs and can build up to extreme amounts that you neither need nor can excrete. Talk with your doctor if you have questions about whether your multivitamin provides sufficient amounts of any given nutrient.

Don't go overboard. Many supplements contain excessive amounts of a certain nutrient—say 433 percent of the recommended daily allowance. Unless your health care provider tells you otherwise, purchase a supplement that contains 100 percent or less of a nutrient and rely on your diet to supply the rest of your needs. In some cases, as with omega-3s, there is no specific recommended intake. Check out ConsumerLab.com for reviews of the safest and most effective supplements.

Can Any Vitamin or Mineral Supplements Aid Weight Loss?

Unfortunately, no. Some supplements—such as herbals—might be effective in promoting weight loss, but the side effects can be more than you bargained for. And these types of supplements are not closely regulated, which means the FDA doesn't provide the same level of oversight it gives to food items. So be wary of any supplement that sounds too good to be true—it probably is. Your best bet is to make sure you're taking in adequate—but not excessive—amounts of B vitamins to keep your metabolism humming along.

If you do want to add a supplement, choose one that's an extract of a real food, such as green tea. But as with all things, don't go overboard.

A recent study published in the *Journal of Nutrition*[3] found that when study participants consumed a beverage rich (approximately 625 milligrams) in the catechins found in green tea, they lost more weight and more abdominal fat than the control group. But do you need to run out and buy a green tea extract supplement? Probably not. One cup of green tea provides about 140 milligrams, and additional research has found that consuming about 3 cups a day is effective in promoting fat oxidation.

THE TAKEAWAY

Eat your fruits and veggies. Those foods are packed with the nutrients, vitamins, and minerals you need. It's easier for your body to absorb vitamins and minerals from foods than from pills. Plus, with fruits and veggies, you also get fiber and hydration to keep your body running strong.

Take a multivitamin. If you've been cutting calories, avoiding certain food groups, or ratcheting up your exercise routine, it's a good idea to take a multivitamin to ensure you're getting the vitamins and minerals you need.

See a doctor. If you're feeling chronically run-down, see a doctor and have your blood tested to determine if you have any particular nutrient deficiencies that may be affecting your health and performance.

14

Adapting Mainstream Dieting Strategies to Run to Lose

I f you want to get fit and lose weight, you've got to make changes to what you eat and how you work out. So it's hard to resist the lure of diets that promise instant, permanent results with little work or restraint.

The truth is that diets are a lot like training plans. No one diet is best for everyone. There's only a way of eating that's the best fit for your lifestyle, needs, goals, and resources at any given time. Most diets are similar in that they involve cutting calories (sometimes drastically) and modifying the proportions of foods and food groups you might typically eat. But within each of these categories, each diet has certain parameters you must follow to reap the purported benefits.

Some diets have a laundry list of rules, while others focus more on simply eliminating a specific ingredient (or entire food group). Still others allow every food you can dream of—but in small portions—or require you to order the meals and snacks from a certain manufacturer.

Other diets are more general styles of eating. They prescribe set calorie limits to help you avoid obvious bad actors such as high-fat, high-sodium, and high-sugar junk foods. Each diet has its benefits and drawbacks for each individual. The most important factor in any diet is how well it helps you meet your goals, fits your needs, and helps you maintain healthy eating habits for life.

Over the years, your own personal "perfect diet" will evolve as you discover what works best for you. You will gravitate toward the foods that make you feel healthy, lean, strong, and energized for your workouts. Foods that leave you feeling tired, bloated, or unsatisfied will ultimately lose their appeal.

Here's what you need to know about some of the more popular diets on the market and how to adapt them to fit your running goals.

Low-Carb Diets

The premise: Technically, any low-carbohydrate diet is an eating plan consisting of less than 20 percent of a day's calories from carbohydrate, or approximately 20 to 60 grams per day. Each has a twist. Some diets call for a most drastic reduction—less than 40 grams of carbs per day at first—reasoning that this forces the body to burn both stored fat and an energy source known as ketones. Other diets limit carbs to 40 percent of daily calories and call for the balance to be split equally between protein and fat.

The upside: The diets are effective since you omit many of the empty calorie junk foods (like cupcakes, candy, and snacks) that are high in carbs and pack on the pounds. Proponents claim that weight loss will quickly and naturally follow restriction of sugars and carbohydrates. And indeed, you'll see results right away on the bathroom scale. When you slash carbs, you retain less water, and the water in your system will be flushed out. Also, because many of these diets allow you unlimited fats and protein, you can indulge in carb-free foods you might have previously written off, such as eggs and bacon. And because fat and protein are digested more slowly, you'll feel fuller longer and avoid feelings of deprivation that can lead to a binge down the road.

The downside: Carbohydrate is the nutrient your body can most efficiently convert into the energy you need to run strong, without causing GI distress. (Most runners should get at least 55 percent of their daily calories from carbs.) The body digests fats and protein more slowly. So if you're on a low-carb diet, you won't feel as energized on the run, and you may have to be more careful about what you eat before you run. In addition, many runners find these diets difficult to sustain. Finally, when you completely eliminate crucial food groups such as fruits and vegetables, you may set yourself up for nutrient deficiencies. Can a multivitamin provide nutrients such as vitamin C and K? Yes. Can it provide naturally occurring antioxidants and flavonoids, and other bioactive components that are essential to optimum health? Probably not.

Is it safe? Short-term, these diets appear to be safe, but research has yet to determine the impact of such diets on the development of chronic diseases such as type 2 diabetes, osteoporosis, and kidney disease. Because you eliminate many food groups when you go low carb, you can develop certain nutrient deficiencies.

Will it work? Based on anecdotal evidence and peer-reviewed research, when practiced in a sustainable way, low-carb diets can work. A study published in the September 2014 issue of the *Annals of Internal Medicine* found that low-carb diets were more effective for weight loss than low-fat diets; plus they reduced risk of heart disease more than low-fat diets did.[1]

How to adapt the diet to lose weight and run faster: Low-carb diets can work if weight loss is your primary goal. But if you're running on a regular basis or training for a race, you'll need to keep some carbs in your diet in order to see your goal time on the finish-line clock and maximize your calorie burn on the road. Rather than cutting out carbs as a group, you might use the principles of low-carb dieting to avoid simple, junk carbs that might be dragging down your weight-loss efforts and ultimately hurting your long-term health. You probably already know where these calories come from—processed, high-sugar, white-flour-rich choices such as quick breads, crackers, and other quick snacks. (Read more about carbs in Chapter 1.) Work on replacing these refined carbs with carbohydrate-rich whole grains, low-fat dairy, starchy vegetables, and fruit. And time your intake so you're leveraging these carbs to boost your running performance. Consume your most carb-rich foods during the times they're going to be quickly burned—in the hour before and the hour after a tough workout. The rest of the time, fill your plate with lean protein, vegetables, and heart-healthy fats.

You might follow this rule: Cut back carbs at all meals except the one before your running workout. Before a marathon, several days of carb-loading will likely pay off, but you don't necessarily need high carbs all the time during your regular training. (For more on carb-loading, turn to Chapter 20.)

High-Protein Diets

The premise: Like other low-carb diets, this approach to eating focuses on replacing carbohydrates with protein, reasoning that the body digests it more slowly—so you feel fuller longer—and that it helps build and repair your working muscles. High-protein diets, which often fit under the umbrella term of "paleo," strongly encourage foods that can be hunted, gathered, or fished and are based on the theory that our bodies are designed to eat like our caveman ancestors; they're not designed to digest the processed foods that are the basis of the standard American diet. They generally advocate sticking with various grass-fed meats, wild fish, poultry, eggs, nuts, fruit, and vegetables—which are generally high in protein and fiber and low in carbohydrates—and avoiding grains and starchy vegetables. Healthy fats are also recommended. These diets tend to restrict certain foods, such as peanuts, lentils, beans, peas, and processed sugar.

The upside: No doubt about it, cutting out refined carbs and pro-cessed foods will help you lose weight and be healthier all around. After all, many of these processed foods include high amounts of salt, preservatives, and refined sugar and offer little nutritional benefit. And with all that protein and fiber, you're not likely to go hungry. Stud-ies have shown that people who eat more protein—about 30 percent of total calories—are less hungry, eat less, and lose more weight compared to those who consume those same calories from carbohydrate or fat sources.[2] And studies have shown that those who upped their protein intake were 50 percent less likely to regain the weight they lost, and they lowered their percentage of body fat.[3]

The downside: Because these diets are so high in fiber, your diges-tive health may improve, but it may be tough to get through a long run without a few pit stops or without hitting the wall. Because the body runs most efficiently when it's using carbs for fuel, it has a harder time converting fat to fuel. So you may feel sluggish while you're adjusting to this new diet. And if you're running longer distances—say up to a 10-K or a half-marathon—it may be challenging to find any sports energy gels or chews that meet the parameters of the diet. And because lean meats (the basis of paleo diets) cost more per pound than most grains, strictly following the diet may cause your grocery bill to swell.

Is it safe? Yes. But keep in mind that this diet is low in many essen-tial vitamins and minerals you need to run strong. And you might find it difficult to maintain over the long term. If you're contending with any kidney conditions, talk with your doctor before trying a high-protein diet. If you're following a high-protein diet, it's best to increase your intake of water. Research has shown that higher protein intakes cause the kidneys to produce more concentrated urine, which can be a sign of dehydration. How much more water should you drink? You can determine that by checking the color of your urine; if it's the color of light straw, you're hydrated. If it's darker, more like the color of apple juice, drink more.

Does it work? If you're replacing lots of junk food and refined grains with healthier options such as nuts, dried fruit, and lean protein, you're likely to shed some weight. Studies have shown that when obese men were given a variety of meals, those who consumed high-protein, high-fat, and very low-carb meals felt less hungry and more full (and lost more weight) compared to men fed moderate-carb, protein, and fat meals.[4] And studies have shown that those who cut their calories to lose weight while upping their protein intake to twice the recommended Daily Value (0.73 gram of protein per pound of body weight) lost more fat mass while retaining their hard-earned muscle mass.[5]

How to adapt the diet to lose weight and run faster: There's nothing wrong with cutting out refined grains and junk carbs—this will improve your weight and your overall health. But if you cut out all grains (including whole grains), you will remove many essential vitamins—such as B vitamins—from your diet. And if you cut out dairy products, you'll want to consider adding in another source of calcium and vitamin D.

To make a high-protein diet work for you, there's no need to go all-out. Doing so might derail your training and your overall health. But there's something to be said for replacing fluffy, refined white bread with lean, satiating sources of protein. It will keep you fuller longer and still give you that dose of B vitamins your body needs. For breakfast, have a protein shake or smoothie rather than a bagel. For lunch, skip the croutons and sweet dressing and instead double up on the greens as well as low-fat cheese and meat. For a snack, grab some Greek yogurt and nuts rather than stacks of crackers and cheese. While the cheese is low carb, it's hard to stop at just one serving of crackers. At dinner, if you're hankering for a second helping, grab a second helping of chicken rather than pasta or breadsticks. At the end of the day, you'll have consumed more protein and less carb than if you weren't going "low carb." Over time, you might just consume less calories and a lot less junk food.

Detox Diets

The premise: It's easy to see why detox diets are so popular. After all, who wouldn't want to follow a diet that promises weight loss, optimal health, clearer skin, and shinier hair? These diets tend to be based on the premise that you just need to rid your body of toxins to feel and look your best. They come in a variety of flavors. Some cleanses require followers to consume specific (branded) beverages for a specific period of time. Other cleanses involve 2-day fasts. There are 3-week detox diets during which dieters eliminate certain food groups or drink "cleansing" beverages daily. Generally these diets promise quick weight loss, healing, cleansing, and a renewed sense of better health. While not all detox diets focus solely on weight loss, the eating is so restrictive that weight loss often follows.

The upside: Quick results; because you're consuming so little, the weight immediately drops off. If you're struggling with weight or unhealthy eating, simply can't get back on the wagon, and need a hard-and-fast break from the life you've been living, a short-term detox in which you fast for a bit or eliminate certain foods (like processed foods or sugar-ridden foods) can be a good way to get back on track.

The downside: There's a good chance that an intense, severely restrictive, or long-term detox diet will derail your training. You're likely to feel fatigued due to too few nutrients, and you may spend extra time darting for a porta-potty thanks to the "cleansing products." While you may lose weight in the short term, these diets don't nurture the kind of lifestyle change and nutrition improvement that are essential to keeping the weight off. Plus, you won't have the energy you need to work out, which is critical to sustainable weight loss. Probably the most frustrating part is that once you finish the detox and return to your old eating habits, the weight you lost will quickly return.

Is it safe? Some serious, negative long-term consequences can come from detox diets. Short-term, you might suffer some unpleasant side effects from so-called cleansing products. And if you suffer from a chronic disease such as type 2 diabetes, these diets could put you at risk for other complications if you put traditional, effective medical treatments aside while you "cleanse." If you're following a short-term detox diet that calls for eating planned meals, or cutting some of the junk out of your diet, there's a good chance you can get the benefits without the harmful side effects.

How to adapt the diet to lose weight and run faster: If you're struggling to get back on the wagon or just need to jump-start a new pattern of eating, a "detox" of sorts might just work for you. But there's no need to run out and buy special shakes or secret ingredients; simply pick a date on which you're going to avoid all your trigger foods. For some runners this might be sugar-containing foods. For others it's soda. For others it might be salty snacks. Another way to begin a detox is to pick a day in which you'll drink only water and eat only fruit and veggies. Like any detox, this type should be short (since you're cutting out some important food groups), but it can be a good cleansing ritual and a day when you won't be "cheating" or eating any junk. It's a good idea to do this on a rest day, when you're not planning a big workout, as you won't be fueling up the way you usually do.

Juicing

The premise: Similar to detox diets, juicing diets call for incorporating fresh or raw or minimally processed juices into a regular diet. Proponents say juicing will make you feel more energized and healthy, fend off chronic diseases, and even make you look better.

The upside: If you're not getting enough fruits and veggies in your diet and simply can't stomach spinach, bananas, and other fresh fruit, juicing can provide all the vitamins, minerals, and phytonutrients you're missing out on. You can get the amount recommended in dietary guidelines and improve some markers of cardiovascular health. While juicing fruits and veggies may eliminate the fiber that our bodies need, phytonutrients found in 100 percent fruit and vegetable juice can be beneficial for the general population and athletes. Juices are also a great source of energy and are highly portable and easy to find. So if you're on the go all the time, it won't be difficult to take your juice along.

The downside: If you're looking to lose weight, and enjoy fruits and veggies, it's far better to keep consuming them in whole form. Eating raw and cooked fruits and veggies will help you reach your weight-loss goals faster than if you consume them in liquid form. Why? Research has shown that consuming fiber-filled raw produce, such as apples and bananas, in its whole form will satisfy your appetite far better than drinking it will. A study published in the April 2009 issue of *Appetite* concluded that solid fruit makes you feel fuller than pureed fruit or juice, and that eating fruit at the start of a meal can reduce energy intake.[6] Researchers speculated that it may have to do with the amount of chewing required to eat an apple. What's more, raw, cold-pressed juice doesn't come cheap. If you're going to juice, be prepared to spend at least $100 for a high-quality juicer, in addition to buying the ingredients required to juice regularly.

Is it safe? Yes. Unless you completely eliminate every other food group and consume *only* juices, a diet that contains juice is safe.

Will it work? If your goal is to increase your fruit, vegetable, and nutrient intake, juicing is a good call. But juices aren't calorie-free, and they certainly don't include filling fiber. As we said above, consuming fruits and veggies in their whole form is going to leave you feeling fuller longer.

How to adapt the diet to lose weight and run faster: The best time to drink a juice would be in the 30 minutes right after a tough workout, when your body is highly efficient at processing carbs and protein. Make a smoothie with fruit—using the whole fruit and peel—and include a scoop of protein powder to boost muscle repair and fill up faster. For other meals and snacks, consume fruits and veggies in their whole form.

Acid-Alkaline Diet

The premise: The acid-alkaline diet suggests that by controlling your body's pH levels, you'll live longer and be healthier. The premise is that in its natural state, the body is slightly alkaline. On a pH scale of 0 to 14, where 0 is the most acidic state and 14 is the most alkaline, a healthy body should naturally hover between 7.35 and 7.45. Proponents of the acid-alkaline diet argue that if you're constantly eating acidic foods your body is fighting to buffer and remove, it cannot take the time it needs to perform the required functions to keep you healthy. Followers of the diet avoid eating acid-forming foods—such as alcohol and red meat—because doing so disrupts the delicate pH balance in the body.

The upside: While not exactly a weight-loss diet, it's designed to control your pH in order to improve your health and longevity. It emphasizes consumption of plant-based foods such as fruits and veggies and may result in short-term weight loss.

The downside: Given the complexity of the guidelines, it's not likely to offer an express ticket to your feel-great weight. In addition, it's fairly restrictive, which doesn't help anyone who struggles with willpower. Foods such as refined grains, beef, pork, veal, canned tuna, fish, turkey, chicken, low-fat dairy, processed cheese, eggs, peanuts, walnuts, tea, coffee, soda, liquor, and beer are considered acidic and therefore discouraged. And since this diet prohibits intake of certain foods and food groups, you'll need to watch out for vitamin and mineral deficiencies.

Is it safe? Very limited clinical research explores this diet's effectiveness or safety. Most experts agree it's probably safe, but individuals with kidney or heart conditions should avoid it.

Will it work? If you eat a lot of extra calories from acidic processed foods and rich red meat and then replace these foods with fruits and veggies, you will create a calorie deficit and potentially shed pounds.

But as for balancing pH, the body's pH is naturally very, very tightly regulated. A change in diet is unlikely to disrupt this already closely monitored system.

How to adapt the diet to lose weight and run faster: Don't worry about whether a food is acidic or alkaline. Instead try to replace some of the unhealthier items in your diet with alkaline-approved lentils, whole grains, soy, and vegetables.

Intermittent Fasting

The premise: Fasting as a weight-loss tool has become popular in recent years. Supporters of such diets claim that fasting can help you lose weight, rev up your metabolism, and improve blood sugar control, all while allowing you to eat whatever you want during periods of non-fasting. Other related diets, which promote fasting or fat-burning periods each week, say that these fasting periods reset your metabolism and help you lose weight.

The upside: This diet does promote the consumption of healthy foods (lean meat, veggies, etc.), but it also allows for windows of unrestricted eating of high-calorie foods. Creating these windows for fasting requires significant thought and planning; some experts suggest that the extra thought process can lead to more mindful eating and therefore less habitual, mindless calorie consumption. You also have plenty of time while fasting to plan out your next healthy meal.

The downside: The diet is restrictive for certain periods of time, and during these periods, if you are sensitive to blood sugar fluctuations, you might suffer from low energy levels and the symptoms that accompany low blood sugar. While you're free to consume whatever you want during certain designated periods, not every dieter has the willpower to avoid eating everything that's not tied down following a period of restriction.

Is it safe? While those sensitive to low blood sugar levels will want to proceed with caution, some research has found that when men fasted every other day for 2 weeks, their insulin levels improved and they were more efficient at managing blood sugar levels.[7] But, as with most trendy diets, there's still limited clinical research exploring this diet's effectiveness or safety. Most experts agree that intermittent fasting is probably safe for most individuals but shouldn't be followed long-term.

Will it work? If you find yourself grazing and mindlessly snacking at all hours of the day, you're likely consuming more calories than you realize and taking in lots of processed foods and other junk. Pausing your intake of food for several hours may lead you to eat more mindfully and make better choices when you return to a more conventional pattern. Athletes who have followed intermittent fasting report that it's difficult to adjust to, but once they get in the habit, they can adapt and function normally. Still others report that while they adapt and can function, all they can think about is food, and once they're "allowed" to eat again, they have a hard time making healthy choices and then returning to the wagon.

How to adapt the diet to lose weight and run faster: If you're game to try intermittent fasting, you should know there's really limited scientific evidence supporting the claims. What makes this diet work is likely the fact that you're severely restricting calories. That said, if you think intermittent fasting is for you and this lifestyle syncs with what you're currently doing, you might give it a try. But try to time your meals so you're somewhat fueled for your runs. It's fine to "train low" for shorter, less intense workouts, but you'll want to time your meals so you have fuel on board before longer runs and faster workouts. And don't forget about recovery; time your "fast" so you can fit in a meal or snack within 30 minutes of extremely hard efforts. If you try intermittent fasting, don't expect it to be a breeze at first. You'll need to give the diet time to take hold and work; aim for a trial of a few weeks before evaluating success or failure.

Commercial Diets

The upside: Some commercial weight-loss programs can be very effective not only in helping with weight loss but also in helping to encourage general lifestyle changes. Some programs encourage people to learn how nutritious certain foods are. They also require members to weigh their foods, which teaches portion control, another important tenet of long-term weight loss. Some programs include weekly meetings led by trained instructors and require weekly weigh-ins and accountability. They encourage exercise; you can "earn" more room to eat as long as you work out. They also include social support online or in person and counseling that research has proven can be helpful to weight loss.

The downside: Some commercial diets—namely those where you have to buy that diet brand's food either in the grocery store or through the mail—can be difficult to sustain. Once you stop buying the food (which has controlled portions) and return to eating regular food you prepare, the weight is sure to creep back. The foods on the system don't come cheap either, so you may see your grocery bill swell. Another drawback: Mail order diets are not designed family style. That means you can expect to receive your food in the mail and still need to prepare a meal for the rest of the family.

Is it safe? As long as you're consuming real food, it's likely safe. Most commercial diets are effective because they enforce portion control. Pass up any commercial diets that use proprietary blends of ingredients that promise to work weight-loss magic.

Will it work? Once you stop buying the food (which has controlled portions) and return to eating regular food that you prepare, the weight will surely come back. Finally, if the diet cuts calories too rapidly, you may not have the energy you need to work out, and that can make the weight loss more difficult.

How to adapt the diet to lose weight and run faster: Some commercial diet plans focus on portion control, regular weigh-ins, and group support, all of which can be effective weight-loss strategies. If you're not interested in signing up for a commercial diet, you can get some of the same benefits by setting a daily calorie target (see a nutritionist or use the formula on page 156), measuring and recording your food, and connecting online or in person with others who are also working on their weight-loss and running goals.

Steve's Story: Designing My Own Run to Lose Diet

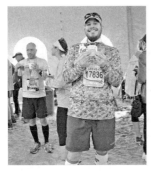

MOST PEOPLE approach conventional diets as black-or-white propositions. You're either *on* a diet or you're *off.*

But for Steve Lambert, the key to losing more than 100 pounds and, at age 33, reaching the lightest weight he's maintained since high school, was finding a comfort zone on a middle ground and adapting a conventional diet to accommodate his unique lifestyle and needs.

"I think with any plan you need to allow yourself to diverge from it," says Lambert, a father of two and transportation planner living in Virginia Beach.

Several failed attempts at weight loss left him feeling discouraged and resigned to the idea that "I am an athletic fat guy, that is what I am," he recalls. "I pretended that being overweight was okay. I pretended that I could just go to the gym a few times a week, and barely doing anything would make a difference."

A few years ago, it became clear that resignation just wasn't an option.

"My sleep wasn't efficient, I was out of breath tying my shoes, and just everyday stuff was hard," he says. "I realized that I needed to be healthy so I could enjoy life."

In September 2013, when his wife became pregnant with their

daughter, Lambert wanted to make a change that would last. He tried Weight Watchers. But more importantly, he took a more moderate approach, using the elements that worked for him and ignoring the rest.

The biggest gain was the education about healthy foods to add to his diet that tracking points and calories provided. And while he traded his breakfasts of hash browns and chicken biscuits from a fast-food restaurant for protein shakes and yogurt, one of the most critical parts was that it allowed him to diet without deprivation. "The key for me was using my daily points or calories on solid choices that filled me up and then being able to use the rest of my calories for my favorites."

Instead of eating half a pizza, he eats two slices with a salad. He can get ice cream, just not the triple scoop. "I always enjoy when a coworker looks at me and says things like 'You still eat doughnuts?'" he says. "I'm like, 'Heck yeah, I love doughnuts.'"

And while it was a struggle to be just one of three guys in a group of 30 at weekly meetings, he came to enjoy sharing his own struggles and successes and hearing about them from others.

"If you don't have people around you that are eating healthier and making better life choices, it is pretty difficult to do it," he says. In addition to enjoying the weekly weigh-ins (on the same scale at the same time each week) at the meetings, he sees "that you can fail one week and get back to it the next week. This isn't a diet. What I do every day is a lifestyle change to eat better and be active."

Meeting up with running buddies for long workouts—and keeping up with the diet group meetings—has turned out to be the perfect mix. With his running buddies, he can get pointers on getting through 50-mile training weeks. "Then I can also attend my [diet group] meetings and complain about how I don't know how I gained a half a pound this week," he says.

And as much as he proudly wears his half-marathon medals, he also treasures the weight-loss coins that remind him of the 25-, 50-, 75-, and 100-pound losses.

"It reminds me of what I have achieved, kind of like race medals," he says. "And it reminds me of where I have been."

PART II

HOW MUCH TO EAT

You may have heard that 3,500 calories equals a pound, so weight loss is a simple matter of taking those 3,500 calories out of your diet, by exercising more and consuming less.

While that's reasonable to believe, the magic math behind your own personal Run to Lose program is a bit more complex than that. A motley crew of factors impact how many calories you should consume on a regular basis to reach your weight-loss and racing goals.

In this section, you'll find all the tools you need to determine how many calories you should consume each day to lose weight and get faster, so you can slim down while still staying energized for your workouts. Plus, we'll offer hints on how to rightsize your portions and servings to help you meet—and not exceed—those targets.

We'll also tell you about the factors that affect your body's ability to burn calories—some of which have nothing to do with what you're doing on the road or at the dinner table.

15

Metabolism Basics

"**B**oost your metabolism" is a popular headline on magazine covers and social media channels. Stories that promise "Eleven lazy ways to burn calories!"[1] and "Nine foods that boost calorie burn!" suggest that if you simply eat more cayenne peppers, sprinkle every meal with cinnamon, guzzle more coffee and green tea, and set the thermostat in your home to 63 degrees Fahrenheit, you can rev up the rate at which your body burns calories (even when you're not working out) and achieve the weight-loss breakthrough you're seeking.

Ah . . . if only it was that easy. Unfortunately, the reality is a lot more complex.

Here's what you need to know about metabolism, the role it plays in your weight-loss efforts, and what you can—and can't—do to tweak it to achieve your feel-great weight.

The Three Ways
Your Body Burns Calories

There are three ways your body burns calories. Anywhere from 50 to 70 percent of your metabolism is determined by your basal metabolic rate (BMR)—the number of calories your body burns to keep your vital organs—your lungs, heart, liver, kidneys, and brain—doing their jobs. About 10 percent of your metabolism comes from the number of calories you burn digesting food. (This is called the thermic effect of food.) It takes slightly more calories to digest protein than it does to digest fat and carbohydrates.

The remaining amount—about 30 percent of your metabolism—is determined by how much you burn through physical activity—whether you're fidgeting at your desk or gutting out a 6-mile tempo run.

CHEW ON THIS

Ever wonder why crash diets don't work? Part of the problem is that they're tough to maintain; severe deprivation tends to lead to bingeing later on. But also, switching to an ultra-low-calorie diet of 500 to 800 calories per day actually slows down your metabolism by as much as 50 percent and lays the groundwork for weight gain, says Seattle-based sports dietitian Kim Larson, a spokeswoman for the Academy of Nutrition and Dietetics. Starved of the calories it needs, the body shifts into survival mode to keep you alive and stops burning calories as quickly as it did when you were consuming more calories. Plus, you won't have the energy you need to go about your daily activities, let alone exercise!

As a result, you'll be stuck in a kind of purgatory where you're depriving yourself but not seeing the scale budge, and you'll feel depleted heading into your workouts, unable to get the calorie-burning and the muscle-building benefits. Even after you return to your normal eating habits, the body will still be in survival mode, clinging to every calorie. And because you've likely lost muscle, you've further handicapped your fat-burning capacity.

If you're stuck here, what can you do to get your body out of survival mode? Most people will respond to slowly increasing their calorie and carbohydrate intake and keeping it under control. Aerobic exercise will boost metabolism, as will high-intensity interval training (known as HIIT), which not only burns more calories than a steady-state run but also continues to burn calories after the workout is over. This afterburn is known as EPOC, or excess post-exercise oxygen consumption. To read more about it, go to Chapter 24.

Factors That Impact Metabolism

Research has proven what you've probably witnessed in your own life: Some people just seem to burn calories faster or more efficiently than others. Some people can pig out with abandon and never feel the impact. Others seem to gain 10 pounds if they do so much as smell a cupcake. It's one reason why weight loss isn't just a simple matter of willpower, or calories in versus calories out. "It's much more complicated than that," says Kim Larson, a spokeswoman for the Academy of Nutrition and Dietetics in Seattle.

These factors that impact your metabolism are hardwired.

- **Gender:** Men tend to have more muscle than women do, and since muscle burns more calories than fat, they tend to have a faster metabolism too—anywhere from 3 to 10 percent higher than that of women, studies have shown.[2]

- **Age:** As you get older, your basal metabolic rate drops somewhere between 3 to 5 percent per decade after the age of 18.[3] Part of that has to do with the fact that in general, as you age, your body composition changes. The proportion of your calorie-burning muscle shrinks, while your proportion of fat rises. Plus, you tend to be less active as you age. When you're young, you're at school, on the go, and more likely to spend your free time physically active. As you age, you spend more time sitting in an office and spend your free time in sedentary activities, such as watching TV.[4]

- **Menopause:** While this is a relatively new area of research, scientists are learning more about how metabolism and fat gain are impacted by the onset of menopause, which occurs the year after women stop menstruating (typically around age 50) and causes estrogen levels to plummet. While menopause may not necessarily cause weight gain, researchers now know that menopause does change the way women store fat. The rate at which women store visceral fat, which surrounds the vital organs in the belly, starts to increase, according to a 2012 review of research by the International Menopause Society.[5] Another study showed that postmenopausal women burned less fat than younger women.[6] That's a problem, since increased belly fat increases risk of diabetes, heart disease, stroke, and even some cancers. That said, there's evidence that keeping up your running routine can help. Studies have shown that women who gained the most weight—and the most belly fat—were the ones whose activity decreased the most. Those who kept a stable weight exercised for an average of 1 hour a day. What's more, those who were the leanest going into menopause had the lowest risk of seeing the weight gain.[7]

Room for Improvement

While changing your age or your gender might not be feasible, there are certain ways you can rev up your calorie burn. They're no substitute for improving your diet. And they're not magic bullets. But taking these steps will help.

- **Sleep more.** Studies have shown that those who sleep less than 5 or 6 hours per night have a higher risk of being overweight.[8] When you don't get enough sleep, the hormone ghrelin, which tells your body "I'm hungry!" spikes, while leptin, which tells your body "I'm full!" drops.[9] A study published in the March 2013 issue of *Proceedings of the National Academy of Sciences* showed that when people don't get enough sleep, they tend to eat more. Researchers concluded that when subjects didn't get enough sleep, they ate more to get the energy they didn't have because of the sleep deprivation. So when food was plentiful, they ate more than they needed.[10]

- **Drink caffeine, eat cayenne peppers, sprinkle cinnamon, etc.**
  Ingredients such as chile peppers, cinnamon, caffeine, and
  green tea have been associated with boosting metabolism. Yes,
  the research has proven that these foods boost metabolism
  slightly in the short term. And while the phrase "fat-burning
  foods" may sell magazines and books, none of these foods on its
  own is going to give you an express ticket to your feel-great
  weight without bigger changes. A review of caffeine studies
  published in the March 2011 issue of *Obesity Reviews* found that
  caffeine intake increased calorie burn, and that catechin-
  caffeine mixtures—like that in green tea—increased fat burn
  over a 24-hour period.[11] Various studies have shown that capsai-
  cin, a compound in red chile peppers, jalapeños, habañeros, and
  cayenne peppers, boosts metabolism and increases feelings of
  fullness and satisfaction so you eat less.[12] Because these foods
  boost metabolism by such a small amount, Larson says, if you're
  looking for a bigger boost, you'd be better off focusing on the
  30 percent you can impact with physical activity.

- **Weight train.** You've probably heard that muscle burns more
  calories than fat. It's true. Some estimates say each pound of
  muscle burns anywhere from 4.5 to 7 calories per day compared
  to 2 calories per day burned by a pound of fat. (See Chapter 25
  for body-weight exercises you can do at home.) "If you have a
  sluggish metabolism, the biggest way to make an impact is to
  increase your muscle mass," says Larson. "We have to be able to
  build more muscle, because the more lean body mass you have,
  the higher your need for calories."

- **Speed train.** The faster you run, the more calories you burn per
  minute. While this might not impact your resting metabolic
  rate, it can definitely increase your calorie burn, even after
  you're done working out. Obviously, you can't run fast every

day; you'd get injured. But swapping a tempo run or interval workout for your easy run is a good way to burn calories. (See Chapter 24 for more on working out for weight loss.)

THE TAKEAWAY

Get some sleep. Get more than 6 hours of sleep per night; 8 is ideal. And you'll need to rest up to rev up your energy, not reach for food.

Hit the gym and rev up your workouts a few times a week. Building lean muscle mass and adding higher-intensity workouts can increase your calorie burn, even when you're done working out.

See a doctor if you're concerned. If you're exercising, not losing weight, and experiencing some symptoms of another medical condition, see a doctor.

16

Calculating How Many Calories You Need

A s with so many questions in nutrition, the answer to how many cal-ories you should consume each day is complex, not straightforward.

If you're trying to figure it out, your best bet is to have a body-mass assessment, with either a Bod Pod or a DEXA scan. These tests are available at exercise physiology labs, many colleges and universities, and hospitals. Because the tests can be pricey and hard to access, many runners, trainers, and nutritionists use formulas to estimate what their daily calorie targets should be to lose weight.

Your Daily Calorie Formula

The first part of this process is figuring out your basal metabolic rate, or BMR. Your BMR is essentially the number of calories you need each day to keep your vital organs functioning; it's the number of calories your body needs to keep your heart pumping, your blood circulating, and your liver, kidneys, and lungs doing their jobs. Once you figure out your BMR, you can factor in your physical activity level (PAL) to deter-mine your daily calorie needs.

When you select which PAL is accurate for your daily life, multiply your BMR by your PAL. This is the number of calories you can consume every day to maintain your current weight while keeping up your current level of exercise.

To lose 1 pound of body fat, you need to create a calorie deficit of roughly 3,500 calories. So if you want to lose weight, you would subtract 500 calories per day from the total number. That would allow you to lose 1 pound per week. If you want to take your weight loss a bit slower, subtract 250 calories per day from the total.

Determining Your BMR

Many online BMR calculators use the Harris-Benedict equation to determine BMR. But over time, researchers have determined that this equation can overestimate daily calorie needs by as much as 5 percent, or 200 calories a day.[1] If you're counting calories, that's a lot!

We recommend that you use the Mifflin-St. Jeor equation.[2] Here's how.

YOUR BMR		SAMPLE BMR	
Height_____ Weight_____ Age_____		Woman: 5'4", 120 pounds, 40 years old	
Height in inches x 2.54 =	kg	**64 inches x 2.54** ········ =	54.54 kg
Weight in pounds ÷ 2.2 =	cm	**120 pounds ÷ 2.2**········=	162.56 cm
Height in cm x 6.25 ····· =		**162.56 × 6.25** ············· =	1016
	minus		*minus*
5 x age in years ········· =		**5 × 40** ···················· =	200
	plus		*plus*
10 x weight in kg ······· =		**10 × 54.54** ················ =	545.5
	plus 5 or minus 161		*minus 161* =
+ 5 for men or . . . ⎤ ····· = **– 161 for women** ⎦			1200.5
BMR		BMR	

Once you determine your BMR, you have to multiply it by your physical activity level (PAL). Use this guide, from the Institute of Medicine.[3]

PHYSICAL ACTIVITY LEVELS

PAL CATEGORY	MEAN PAL VALUE (RANGE)	EXAMPLE
Sedentary	1.25 (1.1–1.39)	You typically spend most of the day sitting.
Low level of physical activity	1.5 (1.4–1.59)	You typically spend most of the day sitting but walk around as you need to and perform activities of daily living.
Active	1.75 (1.6–1.89)	You exercise approximately 1 hour a day or have a day job that is very active and requires the equivalent of walking 6 to 8 miles per day.
Very active	2.2 (1.9–2.50)	You are a competitive athlete engaging in several hours of vigorous exercise each day.

FORMULA TO MAINTAIN WEIGHT		SAMPLE FORMULA	
BMR x PAL =	Calories	1200.5 x PAL of 1.75 =	2100.875

In order to maintain her current weight and activity level, this woman should consume 2,100 calories per day. If she wanted to lose 1 pound per week, she could subtract 500 calories per day from the total and target 1,600 calories per day.

Portion Help

It's way too easy to eat too much of the wrong things. Indeed, outsize portions are a common culprit dragging down weight-loss efforts. The single-serving packages you buy or create with small zipper-lock bags have been proven to encourage portion control. But when that's impossible or impractical, the hints on page 158 can help you downsize portions to meet your daily calorie targets so you can Run to Lose.

Rightsize Your Portions

Look it up. You can use a variety of calorie-tracking apps and Web sites to look up calorie counts of the foods you regularly eat or would like to start incorporating into your diet. Using a calorie counter can help you meet your daily targets. And it can help you make longer-term changes as well. Once you see that you're eating half your day's calorie portion at breakfast, you won't be able to look at that serving of eggs and bacon again.

Measure it. Keep measuring spoons, measuring cups, and even a food scale at home, in your purse, or in your car so you can actually measure out the serving sizes detailed on the Nutrition Facts label. You'll be surprised by how small some portions are.

Add it up. Don't rely on your memory. Writing down your food intake or recording it in an app or on a Web site can give you the assurance that you're staying on track. Seeing that you're near your daily calorie target will encourage you to eat a modest dinner and hold off on dessert. And every day you get a clean slate and a whole new batch of calories to work with!

Visualize it. If you don't have measuring spoons or cups handy or feel too shy about toting them around (don't worry, we understand), here are some cues you can use to understand some common portions.

- **A phone full of protein:** A typical 3-ounce serving of meat or fish should be about the size of the average smartphone.

- **A fistful of whole grains:** A typical 1-cup serving of whole grain such as rice or quinoa is about the size of a baseball.

- **A tennis ball of fruit:** One medium piece of fruit, such as an apple or orange, should be about the size of a tennis ball (not a softball!).

- **A golf ball of peanut butter:** A typical 2-tablespoon serving of peanut butter or any other nut butter should be about the size of a golf ball.

Downsize your plates. Studies have shown that the smaller your plates and the more they contrast in color with the food, the less you're likely to eat. So serve dinner on your salad plates or the dishes you'd typically use for appetizers. On the smaller dishes, your serving size will seem abundant!

Kate's Story:
Tackling the Portion Problem

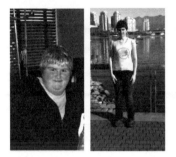

FOR KATE MCPHAIL, how much she ate was as much of a problem as what she ate. Breakfast would be some muffins or a bagel or two. If she was out, she'd pick up a few fast-food breakfast sandwiches.

Salads were drenched in high-fat dressing; bowls of cereal were three to four times the suggested serving size; she would eat an entire medium pizza on her own. And then there were snacks: sleeves of cookies, candy, chips, two or three granola bars, or a pint of ice cream.

"They were so unbelievable when I look back at them now," says McPhail, 31, an operating room nurse from Arizona. "I would easily consume thousands of calories in a sitting by having a pint of ice cream or a bag of chips. I always 'knew' those were foods that should be eaten in moderation. I would talk to patients about heart-healthy diets after they had heart attacks. I just didn't follow my own advice."

McPhail didn't have a dramatic wake-up-call moment that jumpstarted her weight loss. Growing up, she was always the tallest and the heaviest in school and in her family (as an adult, she stands 6'1"). And her family was very active—they would spend weekends skiing, hiking, and exploring.

In early 2010, something just clicked. McPhail knew she needed to make a change. But she had seen coworkers go on formal diet programs, then regain the weight. She didn't want to make that same mistake. "I knew that if I was going to be successful, then I needed to make some permanent changes," she says. "I didn't gain the weight overnight and knew that a cleanse or short-term 'fix' wasn't going to be the answer. I needed something that I could stick to forever."

So she started making a series of small but permanent changes. She started reading food labels, paying attention to serving sizes, and eating smaller servings at meals. She focused on eating whole foods; snacking on dried fruit, small packs of nuts, and air-popped popcorn; and stocking the fridge with fruits and vegetables.

She cleared her kitchen of junk and processed foods. "I knew that if I was going to give this a try, having the cookies, chips, etc., around wasn't going to help," she says. "I knew it would be too easy to eat six cookies instead of one or two."

As a nurse, she understood food nutrients, and she knew what a balanced diet looked like. She experimented a lot and found healthier items that packed a lot of flavor into foods so she wouldn't miss her old meals. She made sure to consume each food group at every meal. And one by one, she started swapping junk foods for high-quality ingredients, starting with whole-grain bread instead of white bagels. "I never decided to eat x amount of calories—I just started to make smarter food choices," she says. "Instead of sleeves of cookies I would make some homemade healthy versions." And she tried to shop smarter. At the supermarket, instead of buying granola bars with calorie counts rivaling candy bars, she bought the more natural and minimally processed versions. Instead of a big bag of trail mix, she bought the unsalted and raw version without the candy, then packaged it into small, single-serving bags. At the constant potlucks at work, she would partake but be selective about what she ate, or bring her own healthy dish that she knew she could eat. And eventually the siren song of the old treats just faded away.

"I didn't look at good or bad foods, but really found that the old foods just didn't appeal to me any longer," she says. "I felt better and had more energy with them out of my diet."

And starting to see the results she wanted on the scale motivated her to keep up the hard work. Of course, there were slip-ups early on. "I would revert back and go back to my old ways for a meal," she says. "But I found my body felt terrible, bloated, and sluggish, and that was proof to me that I needed to focus on the changes I was making."

Along the way, she started running. Though the first day she ran for just 15 seconds, eventually she was able to progress to a mile and started entering races to stay motivated to eat well and keep going to the gym. In February 2012, after having lost 150 pounds, she entered her first half-marathon.

To be sure, the journey was much more emotional than she could have expected. There were the tears of joy she shed as she crossed the finish line of her first half-marathon; there was the deeper pain in seeing, as her body changed, how people treat overweight and obese people. "It makes me sad to acknowledge the differences," she says. "I am treated a lot differently by strangers now than when I was at my heaviest and at times throughout the transformation. I am offered help in stores, and people interact with me . . . something that was a rare occurrence before. I realize that part of it may be due to me being more outgoing, but it is definitely something I have noticed."

Even now, she is amazed by how different her life is from the way it used to be.

"I have so much more energy both physically and mentally than I did before," she says. "My self-confidence has grown tremendously. Many day-to-day things were so difficult when I was heavier compared to now. I remember wondering and worrying if I would fit in chairs or airplane seats or if seat belts would fit. Now every time I fly and just sit with ease and buckle up with many inches to spare on the belt, it is a reminder of how far I have come. Sitting in theaters or stadiums comfortably may seem insignificant, but having these reminders of the progress I made is very motivating.

"When I look back at pictures of me in 2010, I find it hard to recognize that person," she says. "I thought my life was complete, but I am so much happier than I was back then."

PART III

WHEN TO EAT

Yes, weight loss does come down to consuming less calories and burning more, but if you neglect the timing, you could actually see the scale go up and your running performance move backward.

Indeed, when it comes to balancing your weight-loss and running goals, timing is pretty much everything. If you've ever hit the wall before the end of what was supposed to be an easy 4-miler, you know: Attempting to run on empty is an exercise in frustration. And if you've ever had a run derailed by unplanned pit stops, or trained for years for a race that ended with you crouching on the sidelines, you know this.

To Run to Lose, you must think about food as the medicine you need to get faster, sustain an even pace, finish feeling strong, and bounce back quickly from tough workouts. And when you've got a steady stream of calories fueling your workouts, you'll burn more calories, and that will ultimately help your weight-loss efforts.

In this chapter, you'll learn how to fuel up for the road, when to eat, and how to leverage your calories before, during, and after your workouts so you can run stronger and get lighter. You'll learn how to find foods that boost your energy without upsetting your stomach so that ultimately you can fuel up without filling out.

What to Eat Before You Run

It doesn't matter how good your genetics or your training are—what you eat and in what amount can make or break your workout.

What you consume before a workout depends entirely on what kind of workout you're doing. If you're heading out for an easy 30-minute run, you'll probably be fine without something to eat. But if you're planning to go faster (with a tempo run or a speed session) or farther (with a long run), it's best to eat first.

The Perfect Combo: High Carbs, Low Fat, and Low Fiber Will Prevent GI Distress

Each runner's GI threshold is unique. Some runners have ironclad stomachs; others can't even look at solids without feeling queasy. Over time, only you can experiment with different foods, flavors, and brands to figure out what gives you an energy boost without upsetting your stomach.

In general, you want to keep your prerun and prerace meals higher in carbs, which your body quickly digests and turns into fast energy, and lower in fat, protein, and fiber, which take longer to digest.

CHEW ON THIS

Fiber can help lower cholesterol and blood sugar and lower your risk of heart disease and stroke. Plus, it can help keep your GI system in good working order. To get the benefits, men should consume 38 grams of fiber per day, while women should aim for 25 grams of fiber daily. But steer clear of fiber right before you run; it takes longer to digest and could make for some unwanted pit stops. For prerun meals and snacks, choose foods with less than 7 grams of fiber per serving.

To avoid GI distress, keep your prerun meal or snack to these per-serving limits.

- Less than 7 grams of fiber
- Less than 10 grams of fat
- Less than 10 grams of protein

Get the Timing Right

When it comes to fueling your workout, timing is everything. Before your workout, you'll want to have something that will give you a boost of energy without leaving you with an upset stomach on the road. In general, the bigger the meal the more time you'll need to digest it before you hit the road. Each person is different, but most runners find that they need at least 30 minutes between their meal and their run to avoid unwanted pit stops.

If your primary goal is weight loss, it's fine to head out the door for a short, easy run (less than 60 minutes) without having something to eat. If you tend to run out of energy on the road, you might consider a prerun snack of 100 calories. After all, it's better to have 100 calories and finish that 5-mile run, burning 400 calories along the way, than to skip the prerun meal in hopes of netting a higher calorie burn but only make it 2 miles. If your main goal is weight loss, you may hesitate to consume a recovery snack or meal, worried about eating back the calories you worked so hard to burn. But as long as you don't overdo it, consuming carbs and protein immediately postrun can help you recover more quickly for the next workout, so that you'll feel even stronger next time, and at the end of the day you'll torch more calories. (For more on eating for recovery, see Chapter 22.)

What and how much you eat depend on the nature of your workout. Here's a guide.

RIGHTSIZING YOUR PRERUN MEAL

TYPE OF RUN	HOW MUCH TO EAT	WHEN TO EAT
30 minutes or less	Water is sufficient; no fuel necessary.	Drink 7–10 oz, 10–20 minutes before you work out.
30–60 minutes	If you're ravenous or low on energy, have a 100–200-calorie snack that is rich in carbs and low in fat and fiber. If you feel like "training low," you can skip this snack to maximize your fat burn.	Eat and drink 30–60 minutes before you run.
60–75 minutes	Consume a 200–300-calorie snack that is high in carbs and low in fat and fiber.	Eat and drink 30–60 minutes before you run.
75 minutes or longer	Have a 200–450-calorie snack that's high in carbs. Aim for 0.5 gram of carb per pound of body weight for each hour before the run.	Eat and drink 60–120 minutes before you run.
Speed session (mile repeats, tempo runs, Yasso 800s)	Have a 100–200-calorie high-carb snack if it's been more than 3 hours since your last meal. Avoid "training low" for these sessions; you'll miss the opportunity to build your fitness and maximize your calorie burn.	Eat a full meal 2 to 3 hours before you run. If you need to have a snack, eat it 30–60 minutes before your workout.

Ideas for Prerun Meals and Snacks

Here are some high-carb, low-fat, low-fiber meals and snacks that can provide the energy you need to run your best for a variety of different workouts. These meals and snacks are packed with nutrients to keep you healthy. Use this as a guide, but listen to your body. Each individual is unique in terms of digestion time, so you may need to eat closer to your workout or a few hours earlier than what's prescribed here.

1-Hour Workouts

If you're exercising for up to an hour at an easy effort, it's okay to run on empty. But having a small snack or meal ahead of time may help you feel energized and strong throughout the workout. These snacks are also ideal before shorter quality workouts, such as speed sessions and hill work.

FOOD	CALORIES	IDEAL TO EAT . . .	EXTRA NUTRIENTS FOR RUNNERS
1 cup low-fiber cereal with ½ cup fat-free milk	195	30 minutes before workout	The milk provides protein; both the cereal and the milk have carbs to keep you energized.
2 (3-in.) fig cookies	198	30 to 60 minutes before workout	Easy to digest and packed with high-energy carbs, vitamins, and minerals
1 cup berries with ½ cup low-fat cottage cheese	160	60 minutes before workout	The berries offer carbs for energy, while the cottage cheese provides calcium, potassium, and vitamin D—all of which come in handy when training.
3 graham cracker squares with 1 tsp of honey	98	30 minutes before a workout or a shorter speed session	Packed with carbs to keep you energized for your workout
6-oz low-fat fruited yogurt with 1 medium peach	275	60 minutes before workout	This snack has calcium, vitamin D, and potassium to support bone and muscle health, plus antioxidants to boost immune function.

60- to 90-Minute Workouts

Going longer? You'll need more fuel so you finish the workout strong and don't tire out before you're done.

FOOD	CALORIES	IDEAL TO EAT ...	EXTRA NUTRIENTS FOR RUNNERS
1 medium banana and 1 Tbsp nut butter	200	1 hour before workout	The potassium and fluid in the fruit help you stay hydrated; the nut butter offers heart-healthy fat plus carbs.
1 bagel with 1 Tbsp nut butter and 1 Tbsp jam or honey	390	1 hour before workout	The bagel and toppings offer long-lasting energy so you can stay strong.
½ cup steel-cut oats with fat-free milk, topped with 1 cup sliced strawberries	256	1 hour before workout	Packed with carbs and B vitamins, this is an excellent choice for pre- or postrun recovery.
2 oz pretzels with 2 Tbsp hummus	263	1 hour before workout	The pretzels provide easy-to-digest carbs for fast energy plus sodium to keep you hydrated; the hummus offers iron for strength, plus protein.
2 whole grain waffles (frozen) with 2 Tbsp maple syrup	270	1 hour before workout	The syrup and waffles both offer fast-digesting carbs to provide an energy boost; the syrup also offers B vitamins to boost energy and bolster recovery.
PB&B sandwich: 1 medium banana, 2 slices whole grain bread, 1 Tbsp peanut butter	360 calories	60 to 90 minutes before workout	All the ingredients provide carbs for energy. The peanut butter offers extra protein to fend off hunger, and the banana provides potassium to help stave off muscle cramps.
2 oz honey whole wheat pretzels dipped in 1 Tbsp natural peanut butter	230 calories	1 hour before workout	The pretzels provide carbs for energy and sodium to help keep you hydrated; the peanut butter offers protein to help muscles recover.
16-oz sports drink	125 calories	15 to 30 minutes before (or during) workout	Provides fluids and electrolytes to help keep you hydrated. Plus, if you're pressed for time or don't tolerate solid foods before a run, sports drinks can be a great option, as they're digested quickly.

(continued)

60- TO 90-MINUTE WORKOUTS (CONT.)

FOOD	CALORIES	IDEAL TO EAT...	EXTRA NUTRIENTS FOR RUNNERS
15 animal crackers dipped in 1 Tbsp peanut butter	250 calories	30 to 60 minutes before workout	The animal crackers are easy to digest and provide carbs for long-lasting energy. Peanut butter has vitamins and minerals such as potassium and has been linked to lower risk of coronary heart disease.
1 cup apple-cinnamon O's cereal with 1 cup fat-free milk and 1 medium banana	255 calories	45 to 60 minutes before workout	The cereal and milk provide carbs for an energy boost. The banana provides potassium to support your muscles, and the milk offers an extra boost of calcium for bone health.
3 oz deli turkey wrapped in a flour tortilla with 1 cup shredded veggies	275 calories	90 minutes before workout	Long-lasting energy with extra protein to aid in muscle recovery

What to Drink Before You Run

Dehydration can drain your energy and ruin your workout, but so can a sloshy stomach or having to make a pit stop at every mile. So sip on calorie-free fluids throughout the day. That way you won't have to chug-a-lug immediately prerun, which will leave you feeling queasy and prompt you to interrupt your run for pit stops.

In most cases, water is the best choice. But if it's hot out, you're a salty sweater, or you're heading out for more than an hour, you might try a low-calorie sports drink, which can provide electrolytes to aid your hydration, and carbs to boost your energy. Look for a drink that provides 25 to 50 calories per serving and vital electrolytes such as sodium and potassium.

Clearing the System

Many runners feel like they need to clear out their GI system—i.e., go to the bathroom—before they hit the road. That can be a good idea, to help you feel lighter and avoid pit stops. This is where the prerun cup of coffee, which also provides caffeine for an energy boost, can come in handy. (For more on the health benefits of caffeine, see Chapter 8.) Not into coffee? Any hot beverage can help you move the bowels—even herbal tea or hot water with lemon will help. Allow at least 20 minutes for the hot beverage to get through your system.

If your prerun coffee isn't as effective as you had hoped, you might consider boosting the fiber content of your everyday diet. While you want to avoid packing in fiber right before a run, if you have enough in your diet on an everyday basis, your GI system will move more efficiently prerun. Through meals and snacks, men should aim to consume 38 grams of fiber per day while women need at least 25 grams per day.

For more on hydration, go to Chapter 8.

THE TAKEAWAY

Fuel up on low-fat, low-fiber fuel prerun. Your prerun meals and snacks should be high in carbs. To avoid GI distress, limit yourself prerun to less than 10 grams of fat, 7 grams of fiber, and 10 grams of protein per serving.

Plan ahead and leave plenty of time. Just like cramming for a test, attempting to cram fuel and fluid for a run is a bad idea. Sip on fluid throughout the day and give your body time to process it. As for solids, the bigger your prerun meal, the more time you'll need to digest it before you head out.

Drink up. Have a hot beverage, such as coffee or tea, 20 to 30 minutes before you go. This can help move your bowels before your run, so you won't have to make an emergency pit stop.

CHAPTER

18

Avoiding
GI Distress

Aside from being intensely uncomfortable, GI distress can be highly embarrassing and upsetting—especially if you run into trouble and you're miles away from home. Just one bad experience with cramps, diarrhea, a sloshy stomach, nausea, or an emergency pit stop can make a runner too nervous to race or even run with friends, and even panicky racing with a pack.

If you have stomach trouble on the run, you're not alone. Studies suggest that up to half of all runners have this trouble too.[1]

While you run, the majority of bloodflow is diverted away from the GI tract to get oxygen-rich blood to the working legs and muscles, and the skin. The more intense or the longer the run, the more bloodflow is diverted from the GI tract. In addition, the jarring that running involves can further disrupt natural GI function. Dehydration—a particular risk when it's hot and humid—can add even more stress to your GI tract.

That's why it's best to stay hydrated throughout the day, leave plenty of time between your prerun meal and your actual run, and make sure anything you do eat is low in fat and fiber, which take longer to digest.

GI distress has a wide variety of causes. In a study published in the

May 2014 issue of *Sports Medicine*, researchers identified some of the most common culprits and tips to avoid them.[2]

1. **Avoid high-fiber foods for several days before your event.** In the hours before go-time, choose foods with less than 7 grams of fiber, 10 grams of fat, and 10 grams of protein per serving.

2. **Avoid aspirin and NSAIDs such as ibuprofen.** This is especially important if you have a history of stomach issues while running. Both could increase chances of GI distress, the researchers said.

3. **Avoid dehydration.** Practice drinking in training to improve your comfort with fluids on board. Don't overdrink in races simply because many water tables and sports drinks are available.

4. **Don't use overly sweetened drinks or mix sports drinks, gels, bars, etc.** Increased sugar means increased risk of stomach distress. The gut can only process so many carbohydrates at once. If you opt for a sports drink, choose one with no more than 14 to 17 grams per 8-ounce portion. If you consume an energy gel or sports beans, wash them down with water. If you try to chase an energy gel with a sports drink, you risk overloading the gut, which could cause an emergency pit stop during the race.

5. **If you've had problems in the past, experiment with different foods during training.** Try different brands, flavors, and

CHEW ON THIS

Wheat, dairy, fiber, artificial sweeteners, and acidic foods can all irritate the gut. If you're having trouble with GI distress, try eliminating these ingredients and then keep detailed notes about how those changes affected how you felt on the run.

varieties of foods to figure out what gives you a boost without upsetting your stomach.

Beyond Food: Prebiotics and Probiotics

If you change your diet and you're *still* experiencing problems, you may consider products with prebiotics and probiotics. These substances help strengthen your gut, boost your immunity, and ultimately allow you to spend less time running for a bathroom. In addition to providing GI relief, whole foods that naturally contain pre- and probiotics tend to be nutrient dense, containing antioxidants, vitamins, minerals, and phytochemicals that help you get stronger and more efficient.

Prebiotics stimulate the growth of beneficial bacteria in the gut to balance out the blend of helpful and harmful bacteria in the gastrointestinal tract. Common forms of prebiotics include fructooligosaccharides, galacto-oligosaccharides, and inulin (also called chicory root or chicory root fiber).

Just be careful not to go overboard; research suggests that eating too much inulin can increase stomach distress.

You can take supplements or you can find prebiotics in natural foods, including onions, leeks, bananas, garlic, asparagus, soybeans, whole wheat foods, and artichokes. Aim for a variety of these foods every day to help keep the GI tract healthy.

Probiotics enhance and replace the good bacteria in your body that can be weakened by factors such as stress, illness, antibiotic use, and surgery. Probiotics are often used to treat symptoms related to diarrhea, irritable bowel syndrome, and inflammatory bowel disease. The two most common forms of probiotics are *Lactobacillus* and *Bifidobacterium*; you're likely to see them in yogurt and kefir, both of which have calcium and protein.

When It's Not about What You Eat

In some cases, GI distress continues even when you have corrected your prerun eating regimen. While diet in the hours leading up to and even during a run certainly impacts the GI system, certain medical conditions and medications can irritate the bowels and cause problems on the road.

- **Crohn's disease:** This is a chronic inflammatory disease that involves the small or large intestine and causes diarrhea, strictures, fistulas, malabsorption of nutrients, and the need for medical intervention. If you have the symptoms of Crohn's disease, or a history of autoimmune diseases in your family that you think may be related to your GI distress, talk with your doctor.

- **Irritable bowel syndrome (IBS):** Runners with IBS typically complain of diarrhea, constipation, or abdominal pain along with bloating, gas, and highly irregular bowel movements. Some who have IBS may find it difficult to control the bowels and urine flow, especially during intense activity such as running. IBS doesn't cause any obvious tissue damage or inflammation. Often the GI system is just sensitive to the presence, composition, and volume of foods.

- **Runners' colitis:** This is an inflammation of the colon that can strike runners during or after longer and intense runs. The symptoms include severe cramping, diarrhea, and runny and bloody stools. Symptoms can start in the hours after the run and last for days. Despite the prevalence of this disease, researchers still don't fully understand why it occurs.

- **Runners' trots:** If you suffer from diarrhea on the run, it may be caused by diet, certain medications, weak pelvic floor muscles, and just the physical stress of running. If you suffer from the issue, it's a good idea to see a doctor to rule out any other potential causes.

- **Belching, flatulence, heartburn, and diarrhea:** All these problems are common among runners. Most of the time they're related to diet or the physiological changes that happen while exercising. Some runners report that their GI problems are due to prerace nerves. If you succumb to any of these annoying symptoms, give some thought to what you consumed in the 24 hours before the run. Too much fat, fiber, flavor, or caffeine? Did you try a new spice? Some people report that chocolate and citrus causes heartburn; for others carbonated beverages can cause belching and flatulence. It may take time, trial, error, and research to find the culprit of your GI distress.

- **Weak pelvic floor muscles:** This is particularly common among women who have had children. Weak pelvic floor muscles can make it difficult to control the bowels, especially on the run. If you have had children and are experiencing these symptoms, talk with your doctor. There may be exercises you can do to strengthen this area.

- **Medications:** Any prescriptions or over-the-counter medications can lead to nausea, diarrhea, and other GI symptoms, especially if they're new or in a new dosage. If you think anything you're taking may be leading to GI distress, talk to your doctor about alternatives or if it's possible to avoid these particular side effects while still getting any treatment you need.

THE TAKEAWAY

Shop around. Try lots of different kinds of foods and different brands of midrun fuel in order to figure out which ones give you a boost without upsetting your stomach. Stick with what works! Don't try anything new on race day.

Find the culprit. If you have eliminated all possible dietary culprits and are still experiencing problems, talk with your doctor about whether any medical problems or medications may be leading to your GI distress.

Always be prepared. Carry a few tissues or wet wipes in a zipper-lock bag on the run and pin it to your shorts or stuff it in a pocket. If you've got to go, do so ASAP to avoid further discomfort and irritation. Just in case, plan running routes that pass by porta-potties or public bathrooms.

19

Race-Day Fueling for 5-Ks and 10-Ks

Runners put so much time into preparing their legs and lungs to run fast on race day. Too many people underestimate the impact of what they eat on how well they race. If you show up at the starting line with an upset stomach or an empty fuel tank, or have to make a series of unplanned pit stops, it's going to be tough to unleash your potential—even if you're at your peak level of fitness.

For shorter races, such as 5-Ks and 10-Ks, there's no need to carb-load. (Carb-loading should be reserved for longer races such as half-marathons or marathons that typically take 90 minutes or more. You can learn all about carb-loading in Chapter 20.)

At the same time, you don't want to start the race hungry or drained of energy. Here's how you can fuel up for a peak performance and make sure your stomach doesn't undo you on the race course.

CHEW ON THIS

During training, experiment with different foods so you know what gives you a boost without upsetting your stomach and you'll have no surprises on race day. For a list of prerun meals and snacks, go to page 167.

Late-Afternoon/Evening Races

When your race is late in the day, it's important to have a high-quality breakfast and lunch and sip fluids throughout the day so you're hydrated and well fueled by the time the starting gun fires.

Breakfast: In the morning, consume a carb-rich meal with a small amount of protein. Good options include oatmeal with fruit, low-fat yogurt topped with fruit and granola, or dry breakfast cereal topped with dairy, almond, or soy milk. Or try a bagel topped with a scrambled egg, and some fruit. Avoid high-fiber cereals with more than 10 grams of fiber per serving.

Lunch: Midday, avoid foods that are high in fat and protein, which take longer to digest. Aim for less than 10 grams per serving for each of those nutrients. Great lunch choices include a cup of pasta tossed with some marinara sauce and a cup of fat-free milk, or a turkey sandwich with a side of pretzels and a bottle of water.

Prerace snack: If you feel hungry en route to the race, have a snack that's rich in carbs but won't weigh you down. To avoid GI distress, keep your prerace snack under 200 calories. You might grab a small banana, a handful of animal crackers, or even some energy chews. If none of these items appeals to you, reach for a sports bar. Just make sure it has less than 10 grams each of fat and protein, and less than 7 grams of fiber per serving. A sports drink can both boost your energy and carbs and help keep you hydrated.

Morning Races

If your race is in the morning, what you eat in the day before the race is going to have an impact on how energetic you feel and how calm your stomach is.

The day before the race, aim for small, carb-rich meals throughout the day. Avoid trying any new foods. Resist the temptation to gorge on carbs the evening before. That could get in the way of a good night's sleep.

On race morning, have a light prerace breakfast with 200 to 300 calories 1 to 2 hours before the event. The majority of the calories should come from whole, unprocessed carbs and the meal should be low in fiber and fat (under 7 grams each). It's also a good idea to stay away from spicy stuff, which could upset your stomach.

Try a bagel with a small apple plus 8 ounces of sports drink, or an English muffin topped with 2 tablespoons of jam and a piece of fruit. Another good option: a bowl of oatmeal topped with raisins and brown sugar.

And wash that meal down with plenty of fluids. Aim to consume 15 to 20 ounces of fluids 2 to 3 hours before the race, and another 7 to 10 ounces 20 minutes before the race begins. It's okay to have coffee, tea, or a sports drink if you regularly drink those fluids before your runs and they don't upset your stomach. (To read more about the benefits of caffeine, go to Chapter 8.)

THE TAKEAWAY

Do some dress rehearsals. During training, try a variety of prerun meals and snacks to figure out which foods give you the biggest energy boost without upsetting your stomach.

Fuel up with whole foods. While plenty of engineered foods make bold promises, whole foods offer carbs for energy plus nutrients and minerals, without added sweeteners and fillers that could upset your stomach.

Remain hydrated. Hydrate well in the days and hours before the race. Even mild dehydration has been proven to drag down race performance. But trying to pound fluids right before the starting gun fires can lead to GI distress.

20

Carb-Loading
for Half-Marathons
and Marathons

Many runners work hard for months preparing for a long-distance race, then go about undoing all that hard work in the days before the race by eating all the wrong things, or not eating enough of the right things.

The term *carb-loading* is often thrown around and used pretty liberally—typically anytime a runner reaches for a bagel or is looking to rationalize a second heaping helping of pasta.

But carb-loading is not just about overloading on pasta and dessert the night before the race. It actually takes longer, requires more calories, and is more complex than most people think.

Technically, carb-loading is the practice of loading the muscles with carbs in the 3 days leading up to a half-marathon or marathon. The idea is to fill up your body's fuel stores so when the starting gun fires, your muscles are fully loaded but your GI system doesn't feel stuffed. It's like topping off your car's gas tank before embarking on a long road trip; if you start your journey with a full tank, you can go further before you run out of fuel.

In addition to increasing your carbohydrate intake during these

CHEW ON THIS

Given that cutting carbs is such a popular dieting strategy, it can be tough to bring yourself to carb-load when you're watching your weight. But science proves it really does boost performance. A study published in the August 2011 issue of the *International Journal of Sports Medicine* showed that nonelite participants in the London Marathon finished faster when they carb-loaded before the race. Researchers concluded that "pre–race day carbohydrate intake can significantly and independently influence marathon running performance."[1]

days before the race, you'll want to reduce the amount of time you spend on your feet. As you cut back your mileage in the days and weeks before your race, the carbs you consume will be stockpiled in the muscles, because you're not burning them off during workout sessions. And the time off your feet allows your muscles to fully recover and fill up on fuel so they're fresh and ready to go come race day.

Carb-loading for a full marathon is the best way to increase the chances of running your best race.

Carb-loading for a half-marathon is only marginally necessary.

For any run of less than 90 minutes, carb-loading is totally unnecessary, and chances are good that it may actually hurt your chances of running well on race day. (Read more about fueling up for 5-Ks and 10-Ks in Chapter 19.)

You can be as casual or as precise as you like with carb-loading. Whatever approach you take, it's important to take good notes throughout the process so you have a record of what works and what doesn't for future races.

The Casual Carb-Load

In the week before the marathon (and the 3 days before a half-marathon), the vast majority—up to 70 percent—of your calories should come from wholesome carbs. Make sure each meal has some carbohydrate in it—whether that's a bagel, pasta, rice, or cereal. The balance of your calories should come from wholesome, low-fat, low-fiber foods, and lean proteins such as chicken, fish, beans, and legumes. Avoid new foods or very spicy foods.

The Calculated Carb-Load

If you want to take a more exacting approach to carb-loading, follow this proven formula for carb-loading success:

Marathons

7 days before the race: Consume 2.3 grams of carbs per pound of body weight each day.

1 to 3 days before the race: Consume 3.6 to 5.5 grams of carbs per pound of body weight each day.

Half-Marathons

1 to 3 days before the race: Consume 2.5 to 4 grams of carbs per pound of body weight each day.

Anecdotally, we know that as long as you're trained to cover 13.1 miles, you can make it through a half-marathon without carb-loading—as long as you have a few carb-rich meals in the days before the race and refuel at regular intervals while you're on the road.

But carb-loading before a half-marathon will certainly improve your chances of running fast. If you, say, forget to carb-load a few days out or simply can't stomach a high-carb diet in the days leading up to the race, you can taper in the 3 days before the race, and the day before the race, aim to get most of your calories from wholesome carbs.

Here are some general rules to follow for both approaches.

- **Cut back on protein and fat.** To avoid showing up to the race overly stuffed and feeling sick, it's important to decrease your intake of protein and fat while carb-loading. You may be eating the same amount of calories you were before; it's just that a larger proportion will come from carbs, and a smaller proportion of that total will come from protein and fat.

- **Be ready for side effects.** As fun as it might be to imagine loading up on all the carbs you can eat—especially if you've been following an otherwise low-carb plan—there are a few side effects—slight weight gain, stiffness due to muscles being fully stocked with glycogen—you might not find so pleasant.

- **Ditch the scale.** During a carb-load, you can expect to gain up to 4 pounds. Water gets stored along with the glycogen when you eat high-carb foods. And many carb-rich foods are also high in sodium, which will cause water retention. It can also make you feel bloated and heavy. The extra fluids you might be drinking to stay hydrated can also add on the pounds. Resist the urge to get on the scale or to cut back your calories because you're running less.

- **Do a dress rehearsal.** Loading up on carbs—especially if you're not accustomed to it—can feel downright uncomfortable. Many people report feeling stiff and sluggish during the carb-load. That's why it's best to practice the carb-load at some point during your race preparation, in the days leading up to one of your longest runs. If you get used to it during training, it's one less worry during race week.

- **Embrace the process.** If you're trying to reverse years of overeating, or going overboard on carbs, the idea of carb-loading to run fast can be tough advice to swallow. You may be worried about adding back carbs or reigniting a craving you've been working hard to quiet through dieting. But carb-loading is not letting loose and eating all the junk you've been trying to avoid with abandon; it's just a matter of replacing the protein and fat you'd usually have with wholesome, healthy whole grains; starchy vegetables; fruit; and low-fat dairy. And it's the final crucial step to unleashing your potential on race day.

Carb-loading has been found to postpone fatigue and extend the amount of time you can maintain your pace. So if you miss this crucial final step, you risk ruining your race and wasting all that hard time and work you put into preparing for it.

Once race day is behind you and you've had your celebratory meal, you can return to the healthy eating practices that have helped you achieve your targets both on the race course and on the bathroom scale.

Carb-Loading Meal Plans

To guide your carb-loading, take a look at the following 3-day meal plan to give you an idea of the kinds of foods you should be consuming. The plan was developed using data from the USDA Nutrient Analysis Library. Since nutrient content varies from brand to brand, your exact intake may vary from what's listed on pages 186 to 188. But your carb-load will still be effective.

DAY 1

BREAKFAST

2 whole wheat pancakes topped with $\frac{1}{2}$ cup canned fruit (drained)

12 ounces brewed tea mixed with $\frac{1}{2}$ cup fat-free
milk and 1 teaspoon honey

SNACK 1

1 sandwich: 2 slices whole wheat bread, 1 tablespoon light mayo, 2 ounces
roasted turkey, 2 ounces chicken breast, 2 romaine lettuce leaves

2 ounces pretzels (approximately 40 small braided) dipped
in 6 ounces light, low-fat yogurt

LUNCH

1 chicken taco: 3 ounces grilled chicken, 1 soft whole wheat tortilla, $\frac{1}{2}$ cup
shredded lettuce, and $\frac{1}{2}$ cup reduced-fat shredded Cheddar cheese

1 ounce baked tortilla chips dipped in $\frac{1}{4}$ cup salsa

8 ounces lemonade

$\frac{1}{2}$ cup dried mixed fruit

SNACK 2

1 cup fat-free pudding topped with $\frac{1}{2}$ cup each
blueberries, raspberries, and blackberries

DINNER

6 ounces grilled salmon

1 cup wild rice topped with 1 teaspoon light vegetable-oil-based spread

1 cup steamed cauliflower and broccoli medley

1 cup berry cobbler

Approximate Daily Intake

2,788 total calories; 147.5 g protein (21% of total calories); 51 g fat
(15% of total calories); 450 g carb (64% of total calories); 34 g fiber

DAY 2

BREAKFAST

1 cup oatmeal, made with $\frac{1}{2}$ cup fat-free milk

1 medium banana, sliced

16 ounces coffee with $\frac{1}{4}$ cup fat-free milk

1 whole grain medium bagel (3.5 inches in diameter) toasted
and topped with 1 tablespoon apple butter

SNACK 1

1 medium piece fresh fruit

8 ounces sports drink

6 ounces fat-free Greek fruit yogurt

LUNCH

Salad: 3 cups fresh spinach, 3 ounces grilled chicken breast, 2 tablespoons
dried cranberries, 2 tablespoons low-fat French dressing

1 cup couscous sprinkled with 1 tablespoon shredded Parmesan cheese

1 cup hearty minestrone soup with 5 saltine crackers

16 ounces water with lemon to drink

SNACK 2

1 cup raw vegetables and 1 ounce whole wheat pretzels dipped in
2 tablespoons peanut butter and 2 tablespoons hummus

1 cup fat-free milk blended with 2 tablespoons fat-free chocolate syrup,
1 tablespoon peanut butter, 1 medium banana, and 1 cup crushed ice

DINNER

Sandwich: 2 slices whole grain bread, 3 ounces rotisserie chicken,
2 teaspoons brown mustard, 2 slices romaine lettuce,
$\frac{1}{2}$ cup sliced roasted red pepper

1 cup cooked green beans topped with 2 tablespoons
vegetable-oil-based spread

1 medium baked potato topped with 2 tablespoons light
sour cream and $\frac{1}{2}$ cup low-fat cottage cheese

12 ounces fat-free milk to drink

Approximate Daily Intake

**3,357 total calories; 156.6 g protein (18% total calories); 61 g fat
(16% total calories); 554 g carb (66% total calories); 41.5 g fiber**

DAY 3

BREAKFAST

1 cup (dry) old-fashioned oats mixed with 2 cups fat-free milk. Cook according to package directions and add water to reach desired consistency. Top with $\frac{1}{4}$ cup raisins, $\frac{1}{4}$ cup dried cranberries, and 2 tablespoons brown sugar.

SNACK 1

1 cup honey-nut O's cereal topped with 1 cup fat-free milk and 1 medium banana

LUNCH
(Aim for your largest and most carb-rich meal at lunch the day before a race.)

2 cups (cooked) spaghetti topped with 1 cup marinara sauce and $\frac{1}{2}$ cup steamed broccoli

2 slices whole wheat bread topped with 1 tablespoon trans fat–free vegetable oil spread (optional)

8 ounces lemonade

SNACK 2

15 animal crackers dipped in 1 tablespoon peanut butter

1 medium piece fresh fruit

DINNER
(Aim for a light, mild dinner the night before a race.)

1 whole wheat pita stuffed with 2 ounces lean deli meat (such as lean roast beef, turkey, or chicken), $\frac{1}{2}$ cup shredded lettuce, 2 slices tomato, and 2 tablespoons fat-free honey mustard and served with 1 ounce baked potato chips

1 soft peanut-butter chocolate chip granola bar

$\frac{1}{2}$ cup unsweetened applesauce

16 ounces sports drink

Approximate Daily Intake

3,075 total calories; 100 g protein (13% total calories); 55 g fat (16% total calories); 545 g carb (71% total calories); 47 g fiber

THE TAKEAWAY

Do a practice run. In the days leading up to a long run during training, try a carb-loading dress rehearsal so you get accustomed to the kinds of discomfort involved with eating a carb-rich diet. As much as carb-loading sounds like it should be fun, the truth is that the water retention combined with the forced time off (and prerace nerves) can make it downright uncomfortable. Knowing what to expect going into it will reduce your race-day stress.

Take good notes. Note in your training log which foods and carb-loading methods work best for you and which ones don't.

Have a carb-loading strategy. Plan for your carb-load just as carefully as you plan your everyday eating habits and the other elements of your race strategy. Decide whether you'll take a calculated or casual approach, and execute it. Don't use the carb-load as an excuse to indulge in junk you would typically avoid. You want to keep your body in top working order so you can log a peak performance on race day.

Refueling on the Road for Long-Distance Training and Racing

When you're running to lose weight, refueling while you're on the road can seem like defeating the purpose. Why would you restock the calories you're burning by consuming gels, blocks, beans, and sports drinks?

But if you're running for more than an hour and you don't refuel while you're on the road, there's a good chance you'll be forced to cut your run short because you ran out of energy. Consuming carbs during a long workout has been proven to delay fatigue, improve endurance, and fend off that negative inner voice that tells you you can't do it.

And if you do run out of energy before you finish your run (often called "bonking" or "hitting the wall"), it can take days for your body—and your ego—to recover. Bonking during a race you spent months or years preparing for can be devastating.

We hear from runners who hit the wall in a big race they worked hard to prepare for. Often their letters go something like this:

I was out for my long run. I was fine until about two-thirds of the way through, and then I just hit the wall. First I had to slow down. Then I had to stop. What happened?

Luckily, the wall is usually pretty easy to avoid by refueling while you're on the road at regular intervals. Here's everything you need to know.

Refueling: The 75-Minute Rule

For any run of 75 minutes or more, you're going to want to refuel while you're on the road. You want to aim for 30 to 60 grams of carbs per hour, and you'll want to consume them beginning shortly after you begin your run, *before* you become hungry or starved for energy. Bonking can be hard on the body and the ego. And if you wait until you run out of steam or your stomach is growling, it will be too late to recover, regain your energy and optimism, and bounce back. Refueling at regular intervals throughout the run—say every 15 to 30 minutes—will keep your energy levels stable and help you avoid the blood sugar crashes and spikes that could ruin your run or the race you've trained so hard for.

It's important to nail down nutrition during training runs, because whatever works for you during these runs is what should work for you on race day. Determining your best strategy can take some trial and error. To figure out what gives you a boost without upsetting your stomach, you may need to try out different brands, flavors, and forms of fuel—gels, blocks, beans, chews, bars, and even real food. Each sports food has its own proprietary blend of ingredients, and each can affect you in radically different ways.

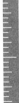

CHEW ON THIS

Be sure to chase each gel or chew or block with water, not sports drink. The water will help with digestion. But because your body can digest only so many carbs at once, trying to wash down a gel with a sports drink is likely to send you running for an emergency bathroom stop.

Experiment during training runs and write down in your training log what worked and what didn't. If you're training for a marathon or a half-marathon, find out what will be provided on the race course. Try that out on training runs so you know if it sits well with you.

If you don't refuel on the road, chances are you won't be able to finish your run. And if you're training for a long-distance race such as a half-marathon or a marathon, you're missing the important opportunity you need to develop the endurance you'll need on race day. It's like, as the old cliché goes, cutting off the nose to spite the face.

How Electrolytes Impact Your Weigh-In

Engineered sports foods such as gels, blocks, beans, and bars contain both carbs and electrolytes to keep you well fueled on a long run. The carbs give you energy. Electrolytes such as sodium and potassium help your muscles work properly, but they also aid in water retention. While under normal circumstances water retention is something we loathe, in this context it's a good thing, because the more fluid your body retains, the better hydrated you will be on the run. (Remember: Dehydration can cause fatigue and drag down performance.)

But that fluid you're retaining will drive up the numbers on the scale (roughly 16 ounces of fluid add a pound). So if you step on the scale after a 20-mile long run—something we've done but would not recommend—you may see a higher number.

Try not to stress about the scale. Within about 48 hours, these fluids will be flushed out of your system. To avoid being upset when weighing in, you might want to avoid the scale for a day or two after a long run.

There's no need to put your ego through a beating when ultimately you're making all the right moves for weight loss!

Match Your Fuel to Your Runs

The longer you'll be on the road, the more carbs you should consume each hour. For example, if you're going to head out for a 75-minute run, try consuming 30 grams of carbs per hour. If you're heading out for 150 minutes, aim closer to 60 grams of carbs per hour.

Each runner is unique in terms of how many carbs he or she needs to stay energized on the road. If you're new to long runs and refueling on the run, start with 30 grams of carbs per hour and see how you feel. You may finish your runs feeling strong; you may find 45 grams of carbs per hour works better. If you follow a high-carb diet most of the time and fuel up well the evening before and the morning of a long run, you may be fine with 30 grams of fuel per hour. Some people who are targeting a PR and burn through fuel quickly find that they need even more than 60 grams of carbs per hour to run their best. Some runners can tolerate up to 90 grams of carbohydrate an hour when they are running extremely long distances. But since the gut can only tolerate a certain amount of carbs per hour, if you find that you need more than 60 grams of carbs, be sure to choose many different forms of fuel and ones that contain both glucose and fructose. They are digested differently and help prevent GI distress.

However many carbs you're using to refuel, don't forget to wash down your carbs with water; the fuel needs to be diluted in order for your body to be able to absorb and deliver it to your working muscles.

Liquid Replenishment

If you simply can't stomach anything solid while running, plenty of sports drinks provide all the carbohydrate, electrolytes, and fluids you need to stay strong. Keep in mind that some drinks have more carbs than you need and may cause GI distress. Stick with drinks that have no more than 14 to 17 grams of carbs per 8-ounce serving. Look for drinks with multiple sources of carbs—such as glucose, fructose, sucrose, or maltodextrin—which your body will absorb better than a single source by itself.

Fueling Up with Whole Foods

For some people, engineered foods and sports drinks just won't do. Luckily, plenty of real-food alternatives can fuel you up just as well. Here are some rules to follow.

Keep it high in carbs and low in fat, fiber, and protein. Beef jerky or a nut-heavy trail mix is not a good idea. Everyone's gut is different in terms of what it can tolerate. When it comes to fat, fiber, and protein, stick with foods that contain less than 3 to 5 grams each per serving. Start there and see how you feel. You may be able to tolerate more.

Consider its carry-on ease. Be sure the food is relatively easy to carry with you on the run. While a bowl of spaghetti might be a great source of fuel, transporting it on the run would be next to impossible.

Aim for 30 to 60 grams of carbs per hour. Just as with sports foods, you should aim to consume 30 to 60 grams of carbs during each hour of a long run. If your "real" foods fall a little short, consider adding in some sports drink or maybe a sports chew or two (if you can) to top off your tank. For a list of "real" foods that meet the criteria listed above, see the table below.

EATING ON THE RUN

FOOD	CALORIES, CARBS, AND FIBER
2 (3-in.) fig cookies	198 calories, 40 g carbs, 3 g fiber
1 small box raisins (1.5 oz)	129 calories, 34 g carbs, 2 g fiber
½ cup mashed sweet potato (To carry, put in a zipper-lock bag and tear a hole in the corner when ready to eat.)	125 calories, 29 g carbs, 4 g fiber

FOOD	CALORIES, CARBS, AND FIBER
¼ cup dried tart cherries	133 calories, 32 g carbs, 1 g fiber
1 medium peeled and sliced apple	77 calories, 21 g carbs, 2 g fiber
1 oz low-fat bagel chips	128 calories, 19 g carbs, 1 g fiber
1 oz hard pretzels (Grab extra-salty varieties if you're a salty sweater.)	108 calories, 23 g carbs, 1 g fiber
1 large banana (Try freezing the banana the night before and carrying it in a fuel belt or a hydration pack. It will change colors, but if you consume it early in the run, it shouldn't be too mushy. You can also mash a banana and carry it like you would sweet potatoes.)	121 calories, 31 g carbs, 3.5 g fiber
½ PB & J sandwich on white bread (1 Tbsp natural peanut butter, 1 Tbsp jam, 1 slice bread)	220 calories, 30 g carbs, 2 g fiber
1 pouch applesauce, original or mixed with other fruits (3.2 oz)	40–60 calories, 10–16 g carbs, 2 g fiber
1 oz hard candy	112 calories, 28 g carbs, 0 g fiber

Rob's Story: Beating the Bonk and Mastering the Bounce Back

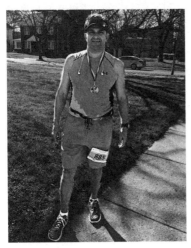

LIKE A LOT OF NEWER RUNNERS, when he started training for his first marathon, Rob Walter didn't think much about fueling up for workouts. The night before long runs he would have steak, potatoes, and a glass of wine without thinking twice.

For long runs he'd stop for some low-calorie sports drink every 6 miles and maybe have an energy gel to get him through the last few miles.

But soon he started to suffer the consequences.

He couldn't run on consecutive

days—even if it was just for 45 minutes—because his muscles were too sore. After half-marathon races his brain would feel fuzzy, almost as if he was hungover. And his longer runs would routinely have fading finishes. "Once I crossed that 18-mile barrier, things started to go downhill pretty fast," says Walter, 40, a chief financial officer and father of two from Dublin, Ohio. Though he took about 10 pounds off his 6′1″ frame, he felt stuck and unable to get that final 10 off to reach his goal weight of 210.

Because the race course was going to be lined with aid stations, he didn't think much about a fueling strategy; that is, until he hit the 17.5-mile mark.

He felt a slight hamstring pain. Then he lost focus. Then the 9:30-minute miles slowed to an 11:30 pace. "I don't remember miles 23 to 26," he says.

Indeed, Walter learned the truth about eating on the run in a painful way. If you don't fuel up your body for your workout, your body won't work. Just like a car, your muscles can't run on empty.

After the race he started experimenting with different gels and sports beans, but his energy would spike and drop during workouts; afterward, he'd still suffer from brain fog.

Under the guidance of a nutritionist (our own Pamela Nisevich Bede), he started eating with an eye toward fueling up for his next workout. He'd pack in the carbs beforehand. And on workouts that would last longer than an hour, he developed a plan for refueling on the road. And no more heavy, fatty meals the night before a tough workout. He makes his carbs a mainstay instead.

"I just make sure that my GI system is clear and not weighed down," he says.

Once he started eating with purpose, the runs got faster and felt easier, and he was able to gain muscle and shave that final pesky 12 pounds off to get within striking distance of his goal weight. But more importantly, he felt more energized on tough workouts; he finished a 60-mile bike ride wanting to keep going. Now he can easily handle back-to-back running days—which would have been impossible a year before. And he can bang out a 12-mile run at lunchtime, then return to his desk clearheaded and ready to work. That's critical, as he's training for an Ironman.

In April 2015 he took more than 5 minutes off his half-marathon time, finishing in 1:43, and placed second in his division. Running that race so fast, finishing his workouts feeling good, and hitting his target paces have given him more confidence. And going into each workout with a clear plan of what to eat and when gives him an extra boost.

"When following a plan, you have more confidence in what you are doing," he says. "That translates to better runs."

THE TAKEAWAY

Fuel up to go long. On any run of 75 minutes or more, you'll want to refuel while you're on the road. Have 30 to 60 grams of carbs per hour. To keep your energy levels stable, eat them at regular intervals.

Test yourself. On long runs, test different types of fuels to see what gives you a boost without upsetting your stomach.

Make a plan. Once you figure out a long-run fueling strategy that works for you, write it down and plan to execute it on race day. If you execute your refueling plan, you'll have a better chance of reaching your finish-time goals.

22

Eating
for Recovery

If you're running to lose weight, the idea of consuming calories right after you've been working so hard to burn them isn't exactly intuitive. For most runners, the postworkout routine involves little more than stretching, some water, and a shower.

But refueling right after a workout can play a huge role in helping you bounce back quickly for your next workout and stay healthy throughout your training, so you can keep your weight-loss efforts on track.

Timing Matters

It's important to refuel within 30 minutes of finishing a workout. During this window, your muscles are primed to take in nutrients and glycogen so they can begin to rebuild from the stress they just endured.

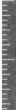 **CHEW ON THIS**

Be sure not to take refueling for recovery to extremes. Lots of people fall into the trap of overindulging postworkout and eating back all the calories they burned and then some. (For more on this, see Chapter 30 on mindless eating.)

When designed right, a recovery meal or snack prevents further muscle breakdown, helps optimize muscle and liver glycogen stores, and ultimately helps the body adapt to training. If you skip a recovery meal, your body will remain in a state of breakdown, and you're more likely to experience more intense muscle soreness in the hours and days following the hard effort.

It's likely you may not feel hungry right after a workout. Most runners don't. In fact, a study published in the January 2014 issue of the *American Journal of Clinical Nutrition*[1] found that running caused a decrease in ghrelin (which increases appetite) and an increase in peptide YY (which is known to damper appetite).

So it's important to find foods and drinks that you can stomach and that will give your body the recovery it needs. Follow these guidelines to quickly and effectively recover.

Get it quick. Plan your postworkout meal before you hit the road, so you can quickly grab it as soon as you get back. That way you can take advantage of that 30-minute window of time postworkout when your body is primed to efficiently metabolize carbs and protein and use them to restock glycogen stores and repair muscle tissue.

Put down the junk food. Any type of carbohydrate will help restock your glycogen stores. But you'll recover better if you refuel with healthy, wholesome choices rather than junk food. After all, if you were trying to repair a luxury car you dearly valued and depended on, you wouldn't use the cheapest possible materials. Whole foods such as sweet potatoes, milk, oatmeal, and whole grains have vitamins and nutrients your body needs to stay healthy and injury-free. Junk foods have lots of additives. A banana and a candy bar might both have the same number of calories and similar carb counts, but with potassium, fiber, and other nutrients, a banana will help you bounce back better.

Make it routine. While refueling isn't as critical after a short, easy run as it is following a speed workout or a long run, it's a good idea to establish a habit of refueling right after every workout so it's second nature when it really counts, after those more intense runs.

Carbs and Protein: The Perfect Postrun Formula

Research has shown that carbs and protein are the most effective nutrients for helping the body recover after a workout. The carbs in your recovery meal restock your spent glycogen stores. Aim for approximately 0.5 gram of carbohydrate per pound of body weight. So if you weigh 150 pounds, have a recovery meal with 75 grams of carbs.

Adding a small amount of protein—approximately 15 to 25 grams—to a recovery meal will speed your recovery. Consuming protein in addition to carbohydrate will help repair muscles and help you adapt to your training. So the next time you tackle the same hard effort, it will feel a little bit easier.

Rehydrate. Drinking after your workout is just as critical to recovery as refueling. Fluids are critical to so many of your body's basic functions, including transporting nutrients to your cells and flushing waste products out of your muscles. If you're dehydrated, your body has to work even harder to recover. It's a good idea to reach for a drink with electrolytes to help efficiently rehydrate your body as soon as possible. How do you know if you're properly rehydrated? Simply drink until your thirst diminishes and your urine runs a light straw color.

Ideas for Postrun Recovery Snacks

When you're eating for recovery, try to consume at least 15 to 25 grams of total protein along with half a gram of carbohydrate for every pound of body weight. Try mixing and matching some of the following foods to find your perfect recovery meal or snack.

Carbs

The following foods have 25 to 30 grams of carbs:

- 1 small bagel or 2 slices bread
- 3 to 4 rice cakes
- 1 cup rice or corn
- 2 cups sports drink
- 1 energy bar (check label for total carb and protein content)

Protein

Each of these foods has 20 to 25 grams of protein.

- 4 whole eggs or 6 egg whites
- 3 tablespoons reduced-fat peanut butter (or natural PB with oil drained off)
- 3 cups milk—choose fat-free or 1%
- 1 cup low-fat cottage cheese
- 1 cup fat-free Greek yogurt
- 3 ounces chicken, fish, pork, or beef
- 3 ounces low-fat cheese (not cream cheese)
- 3 cups soy milk
- Protein drinks and powders (typically 15 to 45 grams/serving)

Jocelyn's Story:
Avoiding Postrun Pitfalls

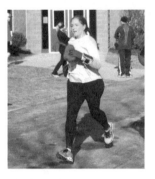

LIKE A LOT OF RUNNERS looking to lose weight, Jocelyn McElhiney was dismayed to discover how much running revved up her urge to eat. Though running helped her lose 30 pounds and get just 5 pounds away from her target weight, she still struggled to lose that last 5 pounds and break 30 minutes in the 5-K.

The biggest problem was the postrun meal.

"My worst habit was walking in the door and going to the fridge the minute I came in from a run," she says. "If I wasn't careful, I could easily down over 1,000 calories without even noticing."

She would grab handfuls of dry granola cereal, cheese sticks, cookies, or chips if they were around . . . and anything sugary. "I was looking for that quick rush of calories and didn't feel I could take the time to prepare anything," she says.

Now, the secret ingredient helping her get across the final mile to her weight-loss goals is preparing her postrun snack even before she heads out.

"I know I'm going to be ravenous," says McElhiney, 44, a corporate philanthropy specialist from Northboro, Massachusetts. "But if I choose my food before the hungry horrors hit, I do a better job of making it about refueling rather than binge eating."

If she's heading out for a run, she has her chocolate milk ready for when she returns. "Maybe I'm buying into the hype," she concedes, "but it does hit the spot and the fluid is filling enough while I work my way to other foods."

While she's drinking, she'll toast some bread and spread on some peanut butter. "The crunch of the toast is very satisfying," she says. Usually that holds her over till breakfast, which is normally two scrambled eggs with spinach and some berries.

But the most important part is that it takes away the panic and the bad choices that often went along with her hunger.

"When I wait till the last minute, I end up searching for a meal while I'm hungry, and that doesn't end well for anyone," she says. "I definitely think mindfulness is the number-one priority with any food plan."

THE TAKEAWAY

Plan ahead. If you're going out for a long run or a speed session, plan your postworkout meal and have it ready to grab as soon as you finish your workout. Make sure it contains 15 to 25 grams of protein. Consume it with a food that has half a gram of carbohydrate for every pound of body weight. (So if you weigh 150 pounds, aim for 75 grams of carbohydrates.)

Act fast. Consume your recovery snack within 30 minutes of finishing your workout. That's when the body is primed to use the fuel to restock spent glycogen stores and repair spent muscle tissue.

Don't forget to drink. Wash your recovery meal down with water. Fluids help all your vital organs function. We lose a lot of fluid when we sweat through tough workouts.

23

Avoiding Weight Gain When You Can't Run

I t happens to all of us at some point, usually when we least expect it. Our exercise and weight-loss efforts are humming along, when suddenly something—injury, a work project, or a family illness—sidelines our regular exercise routine.

When your running is derailed for any reason, it can be easy to pack on the pounds. Some people keep up the regular eating routines that fuel their running even though they're not lacing up. For others, the absence of the stress release that running provides makes it even easier to give in to the call of junk food.

But weight gain when you can't run doesn't have to be a foregone conclusion.

Here's how to prevent the number on the scale from going up while your mileage goes down.

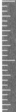

CHEW ON THIS

When our standard calorie burn gets stifled, we often don't adjust our calorie intake accordingly. It's just a matter of math: Decrease your workouts, and you must put the brakes on your calorie intake if you want to keep your weight the same.

Consider the culprit. Where are your extra calories coming from? Have your portions grown too large? Have you gotten into the habit of taking second helpings? Have you gotten into the habit of mindlessly snacking in the afternoon or in front of the TV? Are you continuing to indulge in your post–long run ice cream cone even though you're not running long? Think hard. Be honest with yourself. It may be humbling. But to get back on track, it's necessary to reflect honestly about what you're consuming.

Stop emotional eating. Consider when you might be snacking simply to procrastinate or relieve boredom, stress, restlessness, or any other uncomfortable emotion. Have a list of other calorie-free strategies you could use to relieve those feelings. Post these strategies where you can see them. Clean out a drawer, do the dishes, do the laundry, do your taxes, or just get out of the kitchen and out of the house. Studies have shown that waiting as little as 2 minutes after the "I want to eat" urge is enough to make the craving dissipate. (For more on this, go to Chapter 28 on emotional eating.)

Set yourself up for success. If you've got a weakness for chocolate and you know they're the first thing you go to when you're stressed, don't buy them. Don't even walk down the aisle in the store where they're sold. Keeping temptations out of sight and out of reach—and better yet out of the house—drastically reduces the chances that you'll consume them when you're stressed. Something as seemingly minor as eating from smaller plates has been shown to help downsize portions (for more on this, go to page 158).

Just keep moving. If you can still work out—even if it's at a lower intensity—do it at the same time you'd usually run, so you get the comfort from your routine. And you do get some calorie burn. If you can't work out, try to incorporate more activity whenever you can—get up from your desk and walk to the water fountain, go the long way to the restroom, take the dog for a walk, take the stairs instead of the elevator, or park far away from a storefront to sneak in extra activity. These extra steps and extra minutes of moving add up, and every calorie burned helps.

Get help. Explain the situation to family, friends, and anyone in your support system. Tell them you're trying not to lose your mind or gain weight while sidelined. It will be easier for you to do both if there are no cookies in the house, if the chips don't appear on your plate, and stopping at the drive-thru is not an everyday occurrence. You might get some resistance at first from your partner, spouse, or kids. Try to explain it in terms they can relate to: You can't do something you enjoyed that gave you a sense of accomplishment and some fun on a daily basis. And that would put anyone in a bad mood. If you're not happy because you're not running and you are overindulging, they probably won't be happy either. Chances are, that's something they can understand.

Seek the benefits elsewhere. Remember that running provides way more than a calorie burn. It provides a daily biochemical reset. Studies have proven that just 30 minutes of physical exercise inoculates you against stress later in the day. If you're used to running with friends, it also provides social time, laughter, and connection you might not otherwise get. And just a few easy miles are enough to give you a sense of accomplishment that can boost your mood and confidence all day long. So if you're facing down a time when you can't run, sit down and do some reassessment. Make a list of the benefits running provides, and devise strategies that would allow you to reap similar benefits. Maybe you meet up with friends on Saturday mornings when you'd usually join a group run. You might set aside that time to write or do some other reflective practice that will allow you to relieve stress or meditate. Even a low-impact activity like walking or swimming could help.

Plan ahead. It's hard to make a healthy choice when you walk in the door from work, when you're still shouldering the stress of the day. If you're feeling ravenous because you skipped a meal or missed your usual 3 p.m. snack, making a healthy choice is going to be even harder.

By planning ahead you'll increase the chances of eating right. Try mapping out the week's dinners on Sunday evening. Do some of the prep work (or enlist help) 24 hours ahead of time so dinner is just about ready the minute you walk in the door. This way you won't be tempted to give in to a plate full of chips, crackers, and cheese.

Fill up on low-cal fruits and vegetables. When compared to other foods, most vegetables and many fruits are low in calories while high in essential nutrients, fiber, and water. Aside from offering health benefits, fiber and water keep you fuller longer. Fill your plate with fruits and veggies and round out each meal with additions of lean meat and a bit of whole grain. If you're thirsty, avoid drinking your calories and instead hydrate with a calorie-free beverage such as water with a slice of lemon or a relaxing cup of tea.

THE TAKEAWAY

Expect some discomfort. When you're accustomed to your daily dose of running for fresh air, personal time, and biochemical reset, expect to feel off and extra stressed when you can't run for any reason. Make a list of activities you can regularly do to give you the mental and emotional release running typically provides. Reserve the time when you would typically run for an activity that allows you to get personal or social time or just time outside.

Watch your intake. When you're not running regularly, you have to be extra vigilant about your calorie intake to avoid weight gain. Fill up on fruits and veggies; keep junk food out of reach at home so you won't be tempted to indulge. Work extra hard to use alternative strategies for stress release so you're not tempted to fill up on food.

Address your weaknesses. Use the time off from running to strengthen the areas where you might be weak. It's a good time to start a strength-training routine or start a routine of cross-training or massage.

PART IV

WORKING OUT FOR WEIGHT LOSS

When you first start running, if you increase your mileage and speed adequately enough and give your body enough opportunity to recover, you see how amazing the body is at adapting to new stresses and getting stronger. In general, that's a good thing. It helps you run paces and distances that at one point you didn't think possible. What's more, it doesn't induce the heart pounding, heavy breathing, and intense sweating it once did. And that feels like a huge victory! Which it is!

But adaptation does have a dark side for anyone who wants to lose weight.

Once your body becomes more efficient at a certain distance or pace, and it isn't as challenged as it once was, your calorie burn starts to stall and even decline. Eventually you'll find that the same mileage at the same pace on the same route day in and day out doesn't require as much exertion and doesn't deliver as much exhilaration as it once did.

What do you do?

Don't worry. You don't need to take a leave of absence from work or devote your entire weekend to daylong run fests.

One secret of those who successfully Run to Lose is that more isn't always better. Getting faster and maximizing your calorie burn on the road is about running *smarter* and with more intention. It's not just about going longer. And one of the secrets to getting leaner and staying injury-free doesn't even happen on the road. It happens in a consistent strength-training routine.

In Part IV, you'll learn how to redesign your running routine to rev up your calorie burn when you're on the road and even after you're done. You'll also find a gut-busting strength-training routine you can do anytime, anyplace, no gym or equipment required. And it will allow you to get fit without getting hurt.

The bonus? Your Run to Lose routine will help you enjoy running more and deliver results on the scale and at the finish line that will offer reason to celebrate.

24

How to Burn More Calories While You Work Out

We runners tend to covet routine. When we first start out, the regularity helps us exercise consistently so we can continue building our fitness and work toward our weight-loss goals.

But there's a fine line between a routine that grounds you and a rut that grinds you down.

After you've been running for a while, it's easy to slog along at the same pace, at the same mileage, day after day. And while it may feel comfortable for a while, over time it can leave you sluggish, achy, bored, and stuck on a weight-loss plateau. Even worse: You could start to gain weight instead of losing it.

Why is that? Over time, your body adapts to any new stress you put on it. That's why running feels easier on your seventh day on the road than on your first day. It's why 5, 10, or even 26.2 miles that at first felt impossible to run eventually become doable with training and experience. And it's why running at a certain pace that felt like torture at first eventually becomes your feel-great, I-could-run-all-day-at-this-pace.

"If all you do is run the same distance and terrain at the same effort day after day, you will adapt to that," says exercise physiologist and coach Janet Hamilton, founder of Runningstrong.com.

The key to keep building your fitness—and keep losing weight—is to add intensity to your running routine.

Research has proven that when you ratchet up the intensity, you torch more calories on the road and after you're done working out. A study in the October 2013 issue of *Physiology Reports*[1] showed that runners who did high-speed interval work not only boosted their calorie burn during their runs but also boosted their resting metabolic rate—the rate at which they burned calories while going about daily activities, like walking, working, and cooking.

Studies have shown that exercising for 45 minutes at a vigorous intensity raises your calorie burn for 14 hours after you stop working out. But the key to getting this afterburn (which scientists call EPOC for excess post-exercise oxygen consumption)[2] is working out vigorously. What does that mean? It's going to be different for everyone but generally equal to 70 percent of your max VO_2, hard enough to break a sweat, a little slower than your marathon pace, but a little faster than your everyday easy run pace.

And by cranking up the intensity, you're not only revving up your afterburn but you're also stimulating development of more fast-twitch muscle fibers—the same muscle fibers that tend to atrophy with age and a sedentary lifestyle, says Hamilton: "The more muscle fibers you have, the more calories you can burn, even at rest."

And because it builds your fitness, over time you'll be faster and able to run stronger for longer periods of time. This will allow you to reach for more personal bests and overall burn more calories.

Getting Fit without Getting Hurt

Ramping up the intensity of your workouts doesn't mean you should run as fast every single day. The cardiovascular system adapts to new stresses much faster than the muscles, bones, and joints do. It's important to take a very gradual approach when you're adding more intense workouts, such as tempo runs and speed sessions. Buffer tougher workouts with rest days and easy running so your body has a chance to adapt and get stronger.

It's also important to have a variety of more intense workouts to build full-body fitness.

By mixing up the type of workouts you do—say doing long runs one day, speedwork another day, and tempo work another day—you're stimulating different parts of your physiology.

Take a tempo run, long run, and speed session—a mix of workouts recommended by many coaches. Each workout is designed to work the legs and lungs in a unique way. Tempo work promotes efficiency so you can push stronger for longer with less effort. The long run develops endurance; speed sessions build aerobic power. Use the other days to recover with rest or low-impact cross-training (with cycling, yoga, or strength training), and you'll build full-body fitness.

And there's good news. This doesn't mean you have to find more time to work out. In fact in many cases, you'll get more results with less time.

If you equate running fast with pain and agony, try not to worry. It's actually more fun. Science has proven it. A study published in the March 2011 issue of the *Journal of Sports Sciences* showed that runners enjoyed higher-intensity intervals more than running continuously at a lower intensity.[3] That means you'll be more likely to stick to it.

By making over three of your weekly easy runs for quality workouts, you can get fit fast, without getting hurt. By including quality workouts like speed sessions, tempo runs, and long runs, you can get maximum results with the time you have.

4-Day Workweek

Each week, do each of the following workouts, designed by Hamilton. On the other days, rest, cross-train, or run easy. Don't do any of these workouts back-to-back; that could lead to injury.

Tempo Run

What it is: Different coaches define a tempo run in different ways. Typically it means sustaining a faster-than-usual pace without breaking into an all-out sprint. This is roughly your 10-K pace. (To find your 10-K pace, use the running calculator at runnersworld.com/tools.)

Why it matters: Tempo work improves efficiency so you can run faster over a longer distance with less effort.

What to do: Rather than running 3 to 4 miles at an easy pace, warm up with 1 mile of walking or easy running. Gradually speed up to your 10-K pace and hold it for 1 mile. Then recover with 3 minutes of easy running. Repeat that cycle two more times, then cool down with 1 mile of easy running. If you're more experienced, after a warmup, start with 10 to 15 minutes at your 10-K pace and build up to 20 minutes. Then cool down.

How it feels: While running at tempo, you should feel like you stepped just outside your comfort zone. You shouldn't be huffing and puffing, but you should be able to feel your breathing.

Keep it honest. Every 2 to 3 weeks, lengthen the tempo segment of the run.

Long Run

What it is: Any run that's longer than your typical run.

Why it matters: Long runs build your aerobic foundation, endurance, and mental toughness. When you push your body farther or longer than you usually go, you produce more mitochondria (the powerhouses of the cells) and more capillaries (which bring blood to the heart), and you train your heart to pump blood more efficiently.

What to do: Start with a long run that's about one-third of your total weekly mileage. So if you typically run 15 miles a week, start with a 5-mile long run. If you're targeting a half-marathon, you will ultimately want to be able to tackle an 11-mile long run to comfortably complete the race. If you have a time goal for the race, your longest runs should be slightly longer than the race distance, say 13 to 15 miles for a half-marathon or 9 miles for a 10-K. If you're training for a marathon and shooting for a time goal, you should have one or two 20- or 22-milers under your belt before race day.

How it feels: Get into a comfortable, conversational pace you can sustain and finish feeling strong. You should be able to chitchat without getting out of breath. If you can belt out your favorite tune, step it up a bit.

Keep it honest. Add 1 to 2 miles every 3 weeks. "It's helpful to hold your long run steady for a couple of weeks before you progress—you should feel like you've 'conquered' the distance before you progress," says Hamilton.

Speedwork

What it is: Sessions where you're alternating between bouts of very hard running (at 95 percent of your maximum effort) and recovery intervals. Typically these are done at your 5-K pace.

Why it matters: Improves aerobic capacity and helps you turn your legs over faster.

What to do: Warm up with 10 minutes of walking and easy running. Then alternate between running at your 10-K pace for 400 meters (or $\frac{1}{4}$ mile), then recovering with 400 meters of easy running.

How it feels: During the bouts of hard work, you'll be running near your maximum effort. It should feel tough to say more than one or two words at a time. If you can recite the question "Am I running fast enough?" without gasping for air, you're not. You should be able to say "this . . . (breath) . . . feels . . . (breath) . . . hard." The goal is to have enough recovery to be able to do the next speed interval correctly. "Focus on matching your target pace, not beating it," says Hamilton.

Keep it honest. Start with two 400-meter repeats, then move up to four to six 400-meter repeats, alternating that with 400 meters of easy running to recover. Once you're comfortable, start cutting the recovery intervals to 200 meters. If you want to switch things up, keep the recovery intervals at 400 meters but lengthen the bouts of hard work to 600 to 800 meters.

Hill Work

Why it matters: Hills build leg and lung strength and give you the foundation of fitness you need to get faster.

What to do: Once a week, incorporate into your run a variety of hills that take 30 to 60 seconds to climb. As you go uphill, try to stay relaxed. Keep your gaze straight ahead and your shoulders down, and envision your feet pushing up and off the leg and the road rising to meet you. On the way down, don't let your feet slap the pavement and avoid leaning back and braking with the quads. That will put you at risk of injury.

How it feels: Try to maintain an even level of effort as you're climbing up the hill and as you're making your descent. Avoid trying to charge the hill; you don't want to be spent by the time you get to the top.

Keep it honest. As you get fitter, add more challenging hills with a variety of grades and lengths.

Keep It Safe and Effective

As you ratchet up the intensity, taking these steps will help you make the most of your time—without getting injured.

Pick the right pace. It's important to make sure you're doing your easy runs and your hard track workouts at a pace that's appropriate for your current level of fitness. To find your 5-K or 10-K pace, plug a recent race time into our training calculator at runnersworld.com/tools. No recent race time? Run a 5-K or you can do a time trial. Here's how: Warm up with 1 mile of easy running. Then run four laps around the track—or 1 mile on a flat stretch of road—and note your time. Run 1 mile to cool down. Plug the time of your fast mile into the training calculator to get the appropriate training paces.

Brush up on your track tactics. Tracks are ideal for faster workouts; they're flat, usually traffic-free, and the distance is measured. Haven't run track since gym class? Don't be scared. Here's what you need to know.

- Standard tracks are 400 meters long.
- 400 meters is about $\frac{1}{4}$ mile, so four laps around the track equals 1 mile.
- Many schools open their tracks to the public.
- No access to a track? You can do speedwork on a treadmill or any flat, traffic-free road.
- A "repeat" refers to a bout of fast running. For example, in 4 x 100 @ 10-K pace, the "repeat" is the 100 meters run at a 10-K pace.

Don't cram. Lots of people get hung up on running a certain number of miles per week, and if they miss a day or two, try to cram in extra miles. That's a recipe for injury. Stick to the plan as best you can, but when life gets in the way—or you feel fatigued or sore—it's okay to put the workout off until another day or skip it altogether. Remember: A single workout won't make or break your fitness; it's the accumulated impact of fitness you've built over the course of weeks or months that gets you in shape. But if you try to cram in miles in too short a period of time, you could get sidelined for weeks or months.

Stay well fueled. When you're running faster, and going longer, you must make sure that you're well hydrated and well fueled before you go out. (See Chapter 17 on prerun fueling.) Running on empty doesn't aid weight loss; in fact if you're energized, you'll be able to run faster (and burn more calories) and get fitter and faster. To prevent GI distress, try to stay hydrated throughout the day. Each day aim for half your body weight in ounces of fluids. So if you weigh 200 pounds, aim to consume 100 ounces of calorie-free fluids, such as water. If you weigh 150 pounds, aim for 75 ounces. If you're going to be on the road for 75 minutes or longer, refuel carbs on the run to keep you energized. A variety of energy gels and chews are on the market, or you can use candy or real food. Aim for 30 to 60 grams of carbs per hour while you're on the road. Even if you're not hungry or tired, to prevent bonking, start fueling 20 to 30 minutes into the run and keep refueling at regular intervals. Try lots of different brands and flavors to figure out what flavor and blend give you a boost without leaving you with an upset stomach.

Don't discount your life stress. While exercise is a proven stress reliever, if you start your workout frazzled or drained from your nonrunning life—say you're sick, sleep deprived, or anxious about work—the workout is going to feel harder. Studies have shown that for people who were stressed out, workouts felt harder than they did for those who weren't, even when they were working at the same level of effort.

Take good notes. As you add speed to your routine, it's especially important that you keep a detailed training log, making notes about how far and fast you went, how you felt while you were out, the terrain, the route, and what the weather conditions were. This will help you prevent injuries: If you see that your knee was achy a few days in a row, you'll know to take a break before it becomes a full-blown injury. It will also help you avoid burnout. Say you're starting to feel bored and less motivated to get on the road; you might see in your log that you've taken the 5-mile route for 3 months. You'll know it's time for a change. Be sure to make note of when you buy your shoes. Running shoes should be replaced every 300 to 500 miles, and worn-out shoes are a common cause of injury.

Renee's Story: Working Out with Purpose

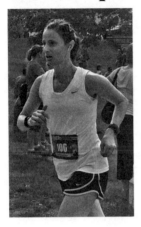

RENEE CORNEILLE was like most runners; she always assumed more miles was better.

"I was so used to equating training with running—and running a lot," says Corneille, a 39-year-old mother of two from Minneapolis.

For years she ran six times a week but only ended up injured and frustrated. She found the book *Run Less, Run Faster*, which outlines a three-quality-workout routine from the FIRST training program at Furman University in South Carolina. She decided to give it a try. When she switched to three quality workouts, she cut her 5-K pace from 9 minutes per mile to 7:21. She shaved 7 minutes from her half-marathon PR (getting it down to 1:52). "I'm just so much faster now," says Corneille, a middle-school principal.

Best of all, she shed 8 pounds from her 5'7" frame, and her core and arms are stronger and more defined.

"Since I started running with a purpose every workout, I'm in much better shape," she says.

Though Corneille was already a vegetarian, once she ramped up the intensity of her workouts, she became more diligent about getting more protein, carbs, and fat to ensure that she was well fueled for each run and could recover quickly after her workouts.

"I was better about consuming the calories I needed to run, but not more," she says. "I was able to correlate the food I was consuming to the quality of my runs."

Even beyond the weight loss, she was buoyed by the confidence she gained from tackling challenging workouts.

"The speedwork was so hard, but also extremely fun," she says. "I'm an average mom of two. I could not believe I was able to run that fast, and it was cool to know I could do it."

She was also able to enjoy her running life more.

As a working mom with two young kids—ages 5 and 3—and a husband with a busy travel schedule, the routine felt much more doable.

"Knowing that three quality runs is what is essential," says Corneille, "I can manage my life and my running schedule with much more ease."

25

Strength Training for Weight Loss

We runners tend to dread strength training and avoid it at any cost. After all, it's hard enough to find the time just to get the miles in. But research proves that weight training, when combined with running, can boost your calorie burn more than running alone.

In a study published in the December 2014 issue of *Obesity*, researchers found that healthy men who did 20 minutes per day of weight training gained less belly fat over 12 years compared to those who spent the same amount of time doing moderate to vigorous aerobic activity.[1]

The following 10-step workout was designed by *Runner's World* columnist and coach Jenny Hadfield, founder of JennyHadfield.com and coauthor of *Marathoning for Mortals* and *Running for Mortals*.[2]

These moves target strength, balance, and mobility, so you can build more lean body mass, torch more calories, and run faster.

"This total-body workout focuses on key exercises for a runner's needs (like glute and core strength, balance, and stability)," says Hadfield. "You don't have to train an hour and a half at a gym with weights to develop balanced, lean muscle tissue. Like running, it's more about consistency, and this program makes it too convenient not to do it anywhere."

And the best part? It can be done anytime, anywhere in less than 20 minutes. Add a warmup and cooldown, and you can do it on days when you can't run.

Use a digital watch with an interval timer and set it up to repeat the interval at 75-second increments. Do the 10 strength moves back-to-back, performing each move for 1 minute. The goal is to keep your heart rate up by moving from one exercise to the next while fatiguing target muscle groups. (The 15 extra seconds allows for movement into the next exercise. If you find you need less time, you can shorten the interval time.)

Repeat this sequence two or three times per week—after a run or as a standalone workout with an added warmup and cooldown—for 3 to 4 weeks.

As you gain strength, you can easily tweak the sequence to ratchet up the intensity of the program so you keep gaining fitness and strength. When you're ready, you can do the circuit in reverse. After 3 weeks, or whenever you're ready, you can change it up again, performing all the lower-body exercises consecutively, followed by the upper-body moves, then finish up with the core work.

Superman

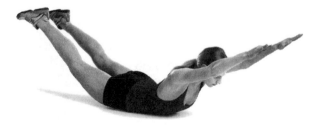

Lie facedown on the floor with your arms over your head and legs straight. Lift your arms and legs off the floor and hold for 5 seconds, then release. Repeat for 1 minute.

Squat and Calf Raise

Standing with your feet hip width apart, sit back and lower down into squat position, focusing on keeping your weight back over your heels. Press and extend your legs and then press up onto your toes for a calf raise. Lower and repeat slowly for 1 minute.

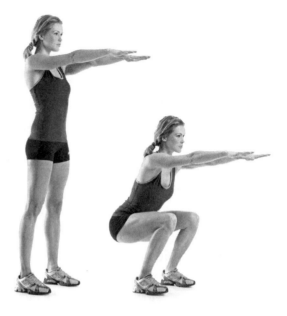

Lunge

Stagger your feet front and back and about hip width apart. Take an exaggerated step forward. Keeping your core in good alignment, bend the front knee 90 degrees until the thigh is parallel with the floor. Make sure the knee is over the ankle and not beyond the toes. Pause and push through your front heel to return to starting position and repeat for 1 minute. Perform 1 minute on each leg.

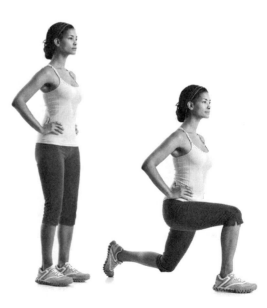

Pushup + Plank Hold

Start in modified pushup position on your hands and knees (unless you perform pushups regularly, on your toes). Press up and extend the arms straight, hold for 5 seconds with a neutral body alignment (plank), and lower slowly back down. Repeat for 1 minute.

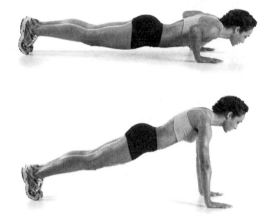

Plank

Lie facedown with your forearms on the floor. Push up so your elbows are under your shoulders and your arms are bent at 90 degrees. Hold your body in a straight line from your head to your feet for 30 seconds.

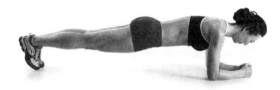

Side Plank

From plank position, shift to your side on your elbow and feet and hold the side plank for 30 seconds. Repeat on the other side.

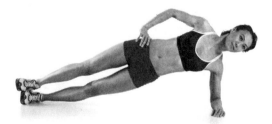

Single-Leg Reach

Stand on your right leg
and bend over, reaching
your left hand toward your
right toes. Stand up and
bring your left knee high
and right arm straight up.
Repeat on both sides.

Bridge

Lie on your back with your
hands by your sides on the
floor. Using your gluteal
muscles, squeeze and lift
your hips off the floor until
you make a line from your
knees to your hips and
shoulders. Pause for a few
seconds and lower your
hips back to the floor.
Repeat for 1 minute.

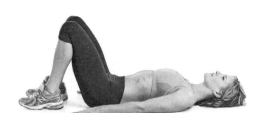

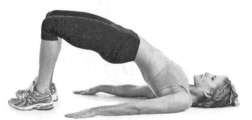

Jackknife Crunch

Lie on your back with your arms over your head and your legs bent with feet on the floor. Crunch and extend your legs slowly straight up toward the ceiling. Reach your hands toward your toes and slowly lower back down to starting position. Focus on keeping your core contracted and lower back on the floor. Repeat for 1 minute.

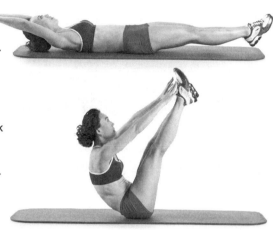

Fire Hydrant

On your hands and knees, slowly raise your right bent leg up to the side, pause, hold for 2 seconds, then slowly release down, for 30 seconds. Repeat on the left side.

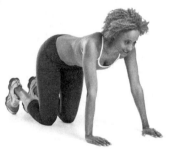

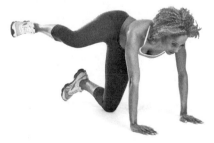

26

Making a Comeback

It happens to so many runners, and in all likelihood it's happened to you: You start running. You push your body faster, farther and start to dream about PRs, six-pack abs, and pairs of skinny jeans. Suddenly you see possibilities you never had the courage to dream about.

Then WHAM! Something stops you right in your tracks. You get hurt. You get busy. You get tired or burned out. And suddenly the gains in mileage, pace, fitness, and confidence disappear as quickly as they materialized.

So how do you get moving again after being sidelined? The strategies below will help you get going.

Get some perspective. What happens in your body when you stop running? There's a decrease in blood volume and mitochondria (the power plants in our cells), plus your lactate threshold falls, says coach and exercise physiologist Susan Paul, author of the *For Beginners Only* column on runnersworld.com. In general, the longer you've been training, the more quickly you'll be able to get back into it after a layoff, she says. So in general, someone who has been running consistently for 15 years, then has a layoff of a year, will have an easier time returning to running than someone who has been running a year, then is off for a year. Why is that? The longer you've been running, the bigger your foundation of aerobic strength, says Paul. You'll have a much higher level of mitochondria to produce energy, more red blood cells to deliver oxygen to the running muscles, and more metabolic enzymes than someone who just started working out. So while your fitness falls during a layoff, it won't fall as low as if you had just begun running, since you're starting at a much higher fitness level.

Also, you lose conditioning in your muscles, tendons, ligaments, and connective tissues. It's difficult to assess how much conditioning you lose or how quickly you lose it. But it's the weakness in the musculoskeletal system that causes so many people to get injured when they return to running. This is why running slower, reducing mileage, and allowing rest and recovery days are so important.

Walk before you run. Before returning to running, you should be able to walk for at least 45 minutes (without pain if returning from an injury), says Paul. Walking reconditions soft tissue (muscles, tendons, ligaments, fascia, connective tissue), preparing them for the more rigorous demands of running, she says.

Start where you are. Don't just pick up where you left off, or at a level of weekly mileage that you had in the past. Too many times a race prompts runners to do more than they ought to too soon after injury, and they end up sidelined even longer. Even if you've been cycling, swimming, or doing other cross-training to maintain your aerobic fitness, remember that depending on the injury and the length of the layoff, it can take weeks or even months for your muscles, tendons, bones, and ligaments to get strong enough to handle running again.

At first, stick with short, easy runs and take walk breaks. Start with three or four short runs per week so you're running every other day. Try 5 to 10 minutes of running at a time, or alternate between running and walking. When starting after a long break, let your body adapt to the stress of a workout before you start adding more stresses. Use the following guide from Paul.

IF YOU'RE OFF . . .	START RIGHT HERE
1 week or less	Pick up your plan where you left off
Up to 10 days	Start running 70% of previous mileage
15 to 30 days	Start running 60% of previous mileage
30 days to 3 months	Start running 50% of previous mileage
3 months	Start from scratch

Remember the 10 percent rule. If you've been off for 3 months or more, don't increase your weekly mileage or pace by more than 10 percent, week over week. Increase it less if you need to.

Stay safe. You might consider not hitting the road again right away, says Paul. The track allows you to walk or run without getting too far from your car in the event that you need to stop. It's a controlled, confined, flat, traffic-free area for a workout. Starting on the treadmill can be helpful too. The surface is forgiving, and you can control the pace and incline to suit your needs.

Don't overmedicate. Over-the-counter painkillers might make you feel better in the short term, but they can mask pain that tells you that you should stop. And for some, they can lead to gastric distress. If you can't run through pain, don't run. Walk or rest instead.

Cross-train. Working out every day will help speed up your cardio-vascular fitness. But that doesn't mean you need to run. Add 2 or 3 days of cross-training to your routine. Check in with your doctor to make sure the particular mode of working out—cycling, rowing on a machine, swimming, or using an elliptical trainer—doesn't worsen any injury. Also, yoga, Pilates, weight training, and core exercises can help you get stronger. That said, if you have done no exercise at all for 3 months, wait for 2 to 3 months before you cross-train; take rest days between your runs instead. That will ensure that your aerobic system gets enough recovery between workouts.

THE TAKEAWAY

Practice patience. Rushing back to the routine you maintained before your injury is a surefire way to reinjure yourself, and even cause new injuries. Don't increase your mileage by more than 10 percent from week to week.

Mix it up. Cross-train with other forms of exercise that work other parts of your body, don't aggravate your injury, and give you a cardiovascular workout. Consult your doctor or a physical therapist about which modes of exercise are safe and smart, given your past injuries.

Be safe, not sorry. As difficult as it can be to rest when you'd rather run, remember that the conservative approach you take now will yield many happy and healthy miles down the road. If you restart your running, and start to feel twinges of your old injury, it's best to take a rest day, or do another activity.

CHAPTER

27

Setting Smart Goals: Designing Your Workout Life to Set Yourself Up for Success

Goals are critical. They drive us to be our best. They get us out of bed when we'd rather stay in; they help keep our fitness on track when it would be easy to make excuses and allow laziness into our routine.

But if your goals are going to help you unleash your potential, they've got to be the right fit for you. If you have a goal that isn't the right fit for your lifestyle, temperament, or schedule, injury and disappointment are all but assured. Here's how to set a goal that will set you up for success.

Make it personal. When it comes to choosing a goal, whether it's a certain distance, a finishing time, an ideal number on the scale, or even what your abs should look like, make sure the goal is relevant and personally meaningful to you. Don't get swept up in what seems trendy or what everybody else seems to be doing.

In our culture, many powerful influences tell us what our goals should be. Magazine covers and celebrities provide ideals for what our bodies should look like. We draw inspiration and motivation from friends' and family's athletic accomplishments.

In recent years, half-marathons and marathons have become wildly popular. It's tempting to feel like if you run, you have to go the distance. But these endurance events are not for everyone. If a goal is not in sync with your fitness or experience, or most importantly, what you enjoy, you're setting yourself up for injury and burnout. Remember, a race takes just a day, but the training consumes months of your life and impacts your work and family lives. If you're going to invest that kind of time and energy, make sure it's what you want.

How-to: Think about the kinds of distances and workouts you enjoy most and pick an event and a goal that will allow you to spend most of your time running that distance. If you want to target a half-marathon, it's best to have at least 6 months of regular running experience before you start out. If you want to run a marathon, it's best to have at least a year under your belt. In terms of picking a realistic finish time, you've got to start where you are. Do a 5-K and plug your time into any of the many online fitness calculators.

Make sure the training fits your schedule. Whatever distance you intend to race, be sure you have the time to train for it. If you're training for a long distance, you'll need 1 to 4 hours at least once a week for an endurance-building long, slow, distance run. And with most standard training plans, you'll need to run at least 5 days a week, plus make time for recovery, sleep, and strength training.

If your schedule already feels jam-packed with work and family commitments, you might consider targeting a different goal. If the training begins to interfere too much with sleep, work, or time with your family, there's a good chance you're going to burn out or give up before you reach the starting line.

How-to: Look at some standard training schedules for the distance you're considering. Map out how and when you'd do each workout on each day of the week. Talk to your spouse, partner, kids, and boss to let them know you're considering training for an event and discuss how and when you'd fit the training in. If your first choice for a goal isn't going to work, target a different distance. You can build your fitness by racing at any distance. Racing 5-Ks will help you build speed so you can kick to the finish; targeting 10-Ks and half-marathons will help you learn how to sustain a faster pace for a longer distance. All those skills will help you ultimately in longer-distance events.

Let the body be the boss. If you've made the mistake of overtraining, you know you can't just beat your body into submission. There's a huge difference between the general muscle soreness that goes along with pushing your body farther than it has gone before and the sharp, shooting, persistent pains that go along with injury. Each individual has his or her own unique orthopedic threshold—that is, how many miles and how much intensity he or she can handle before the body breaks down. This threshold is determined by age, genetics, gender, anatomy, biomechanics, history of injury, experience, and a variety of other factors. And it changes as we age and as we get more miles on our bodies. Trying to train through pain will only turn short-term injuries into long-term problems that will haunt you for life.

How-to: Consider what types of workouts and distances you can do without pain. Do cross-training and strength training help? Pick a distance and a goal that allows you to train within your pain-free sweet spot.

Get to the starting line with four goals. Even if your training goes perfectly, anything can happen on race day. If your satisfaction with your event is entirely contingent on reaching a single time goal, you're setting yourself up for upset. It's important to have four goals at the starting line: a goal for the ideal day, a goal you'd be happy with, a goal just to finish, and a process goal. Process goals don't have anything to do with the outcome of the race. They have to do with the things you'll do during the race to help increase your chances of reaching your goal time. You might aim to execute your fueling strategy perfectly, not walk up the hills, or even run a negative split (do the second half of the race faster than the first half).

How-to: To figure out a realistic time target, schedule a tune-up race 2 to 4 weeks before your goal event to test your level of fitness. Plug your finishing time into an online training calculator to figure out a realistic goal for your big event. Aim for that result—not the time you targeted when you first started training. Training requires months of preparation, and anything can happen during that time—work, injuries, and family commitments can all impact that original goal. You have to start each race where you are!

Think beyond the finish line. When you're training for an event, the preparation gets so intense and takes so long, it's easy to get consumed by the result and to feel a little lost after it's all over. That's natural.

How-to: Schedule a race of a shorter distance or a vacation or a big event in the weeks following your big racing event. That way, no matter what the race result, you'll have something to look forward to after you finish!

Wesley's Story: Why Making a Breakthrough Takes a Measured Approach

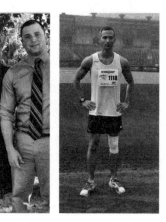

WHEN WESLEY CURE weighed in at an all-time high of 225 pounds and could no longer fit into his pants, he knew something had to change.

And his weight-loss efforts got off to a blazing start.

While working as a deputy disbursing officer with the US Air Force, he was able to get downsized portions of rice, lean meats, and veggies at the dining facility. He diligently resisted the ice cream, cakes, and pies that were constantly offered as morale boosters. He started getting more sleep, which helped him recover from tough workouts.

He was just as disciplined with his running. He started with a 3-mile morning run a few times a week, then purchased a watch GPS and progressed to speedwork, tempo work, and long runs.

Within 6 weeks, he dropped 12 pounds. Then he set his sights on his high school weight of 155.

"I knew if I could maintain the lifestyle changes I had made, I would reach my goal eventually," says Cure, 31, of Bloomington, Indiana.

And his diligence paid off in short order. By September he had reached his goal weight. What's more, he was winning 5-K races and finished his first marathon in 3:10.

But he also learned a lesson a lot of runners do the hard way: You can't go all-out all the time—with running or dieting.

"For a long time, I was running 80 percent of my runs at very close to max effort," he says. "While I saw some serious gains, it always led to injury or overtraining."

First he had a bout of runner's knee, which sidelined him for weeks. "It was very clear that I had done too much too soon," he says. As a result, he started strictly adhering to the 10 percent rule, increasing his mileage by no more than 10 percent week after week. It took longer to resist going all-out on every run. During marathon training, "I was blasting most of my runs and setting PRs every couple of weeks," he says. "I thought everything was going fine."

Midway through training, he won a 15-K race. But the next day he struggled to maintain his typical 7-minute miles—more than a minute slower than his race pace. "I chalked it up to sore legs, but it lasted about 4 weeks," he says. "I had clearly pushed too hard, and my body revolted."

Gradually he recovered and started taking most of his mileage at a much easier pace, targeting just a few workouts each week to go hard. "I have worked very hard to realize that I can stay healthy and still improve by holding back."

He also realized he needed to take that moderation to his approach to eating.

After months of swearing off sweets, "I ended up bingeing once and realized there was no way I could go without these things," he says. "By having them every once in a while, I avoid those incidents. Sure, it is fine to forgo during certain parts of my marathon-specific portion of training, but to try to give up the occasional sweets and greasy meal just wasn't realistic for me. So I eat a little so I don't want a lot."

PART V

WHY WE EAT

While supersize portions and junk food are surely major obstacles to weight loss, some of the biggest obstacles often have nothing to do with nutrition content or serving size. For many people, the emotional, mental, and environmental forces that drive them to eat are among the major problems.

If you've ever been cheered up by a sweet treat or found yourself powerless in the face of your child's bag of Halloween candy, you know: Often our reasons for eating have nothing to do with food.

At first glance, this can be daunting; after all, emotional eating habits aren't something we can change by simply ordering something different at a restaurant or serving dinner on a smaller plate. Often we don't have control over the work, family, and other life stresses that drive us to eat. And we often can't control how much and what kinds of foods our colleagues leave in the office break room or that we encounter while we're waiting to check out at the gas station.

But there's good news.

By learning how intense emotions and environmental triggers shape our eating habits, we can design our personal Run to Lose programs to make lasting changes and develop healthier habits that set us up for success. In the next section, you'll learn how to do that.

CHAPTER

28

Emotional Eating

Often when we say "I'm hungry," what we really mean is that we're longing for something else—relief for some other uncomfortable sensation, such as boredom, stress, loneliness, fear, anger, sadness, shock, depression, disappointment, or even a high-charged sense of elation.

In our culture, we are accustomed to getting instant gratification for our every desire and easy escapes from even the slightest tinge of emotional discomfort.

While substances such as alcohol and cigarettes and illicit ones such as drugs offer quick and easy ways to numb out those discomforts, most people find that such substances are not so compatible with their work, family, and running lives. After all, if you're meeting your buddies for that 6 a.m. long run Sunday morning, you can't risk a hangover by partying hard on Saturday night.

Given how cheap and available unhealthy foods are and how many marketing vehicles are out there enticing us to reach for them (which we'll address in Chapter 30), it only makes sense that anyone—even weight-conscious runners—will use food to anesthetize themselves from emotional discomfort.

Unhealthy snacks—from candy bars to muffins to fast food—are an easy, accessible, cheap, legal, and socially acceptable form of self-medication.

Compounding the problem: The sugar that many of these sweet treats contain has been scientifically proven to be addictive. Studies have shown that sugar ignites cravings, tolerance, and withdrawal just like drugs do. In a July 2013 issue of *Current Opinion in Clinical Nutrition and Metabolic Care*,[1] researchers concluded that "sugar and sweet reward can not only substitute to addictive drugs, such as cocaine, but can even be more rewarding and attractive."

(You can read more about sugar in Chapter 4.)

Given how addictive so many sweet treats are, and how tightly food is yoked to comfort in our culture, it's often difficult to distinguish between a growling stomach and an emotional hunger for something that can't be satisfied with food.

"It can be very confusing to sort out the signals and determine—is it hunger or is it emotion?" concedes Susan Albers, Cleveland Clinic psychologist and author of seven books, including the *New York Times* bestselling *Eat.Q.: Unlock the Weight-Loss Power of Emotional Intelligence.*

The problem is, because sweet treats are not actual solutions or remedies for emotional problems—a cookie cannot actually erase your stressors or your loneliness—no amount or type of food will ever offer a sense of satisfaction. Once the momentary pleasure you get from that chocolate chip cookie fades, the stress and the loneliness are still there. And more often than not, the original problem is compounded by the guilt you have for indulging in a sweet that is off your diet.

Luckily, we're living in a time when researchers such as Albers have spent years studying the emotional drivers that shape what and how we eat. Albers suggests trying these strategies to determine what emotional drivers are influencing your eating habits, creating obstacles to reaching your weight-loss and training goals, and how to overcome them.

Question the urge to eat. First, just entertain the possibility that the urge to eat could be driven by something other than physical hunger. Some people will keep a journal and rank how hungry they are on a scale of 1 to 10 or take detailed notes about how physically hungry or emotionally uncomfortable they are. Is your stomach grumbling? Has your energy plummeted? Do you feel like you need a nap? Are you feeling stressed, angry, sad, or lonely? By keeping a journal, "you'll find that there's a pattern for both your emotions and your physical hunger," says Albers. You may have a habit, for instance, of always hitting the vending machine at work for a sweet treat after the daily 10 a.m. staff meeting, even though you ate breakfast just 2 hours earlier. If you keep a journal, you may find that your stomach isn't actually growling for food, but the meeting increases your stress level because you start to think about all the work you have to do; you feel the need to change your physical state so you can get temporarily distracted from that stress.

Wait 2 minutes. Next time you have the urge to eat—or you see your arm reaching into the cabinet without even having made the conscious decision to eat—rather than trying to wrestle the urge to the ground right then and there, give yourself permission to eat after 2 minutes pass. By creating this gap between the urge or thought and the deed, you're interrupting the momentum that leads so many of us to feel hijacked by our cravings. Suddenly we're on the couch, having emptied a family-size bag of potato chips before we even know what hit us. That gap "allows you to explore what's happening," says Albers. It gives you the chance to ask, "Is it emotion? Or is it physical?" Literally just pause and ask yourself, "Am I really hungry?" "The thought 'I want to eat' and immediately answering that [by eating] is so reflexive," says Albers. "Slowing that down does amazing things." The urge to eat can be powerful, and just 2 minutes can feel like an eternity to wait to satisfy it. You may need to distract yourself by turning on the TV, walking outside, cleaning the dishes, taking a shower, or just leaving the room. "If you can distract yourself for a minute or two and engage in something else, chances are you might just forget about it," says Albers.

Understand the difference between hunger and a craving. If you're really starving, you'll eat anything: celery, arugula, meat loaf. If you're longing for something to fulfill an emotional need—something crunchy, sweet, smooth, creamy, or chocolate—it's more than likely just a craving born out of habit or the association of that food or eating experience with a feeling of comfort. "When you feel like you've just got to have barbecue chips—not just potato chips," it's likely a craving, says Albers. "When you're really hungry, there are a lot of things that could fill that need."

Be mindful of your body. Are you standing in front of the refrigerator in a daze? Scanning the pantry restlessly? Picking food up and putting it in your mouth like a zombie? Zoning out? "If you're feeling a little bit almost numb, shift back into the moment and pay attention to what you're thinking and feeling," says Albers. "If you just can't get a sense of what it is that you want, often that's a clear sign of emotional eating."

Taking the following steps will help you pause, think about what you're eating, and feel more satisfied from whatever you eat.

Sit down. Taking the time to find a place to sit down and eat will help create a gap between the urge to eat and the act of consuming food. It will give you a chance to consider what emotions may be driving your urge to eat.

Slowly chew. When you slow down, you make the experience of eating—whether you're having chocolate or eating an apple—last longer and feel more enjoyable. You also give your body a chance to register feelings of fullness. Using your nondominant hand can reduce how much you consume. It disrupts the automatic process of hand-to-mouth feeding that doesn't require thought.

Savor what you're eating. When you think about the smell, taste, texture, and all the sensations that go along with whatever you're eating, you're more likely to enjoy it more and remember it later. You lower that feeling of deprivation that can ultimately lead to bingeing down the road. A study in the August 2011 issue of *Appetite* found that when people focused on the sensory characteristics of their food, they ate less later.[2]

Be aware of entitlement eating. Often people eat out of a sense of reward for all the hard work they did on the road. This is where a lot of runners go wrong. They overcompensate with calories postworkout. In a study published in the May 2014 issue of *Marketing Letters,*[3] Brian Wansink, director of Cornell University's Food and Brand Lab, tested this dynamic in his research. He had two groups of people take a 2-kilometer walk around a lake. One group was told the walk was exercise; for the other group it was a "scenic walk." Those who "exercised" ate 35 percent more chocolate pudding afterward than those who went on a "scenic walk." "Just be aware of the idea that there could be a sense of deserving this," says Albers. Yes, you need quality recovery food to bounce back for your next workout. (See Chapter 22 to learn more about eating for recovery.) "Take a good hard look at what you're saying to yourself," she adds. Plan ahead for what kinds of refueling foods would be good, rather than just eating whatever you want. How to avoid this? Adjust your attitude about your workout. Or even adjust your workout. If your run doesn't feel like torture, you're less likely to pamper yourself with calories after it's done. Download podcasts or movies for entertainment. Or make a date to work out with friends so it doubles as a social hour. If you enjoyed your workout, you'll be much less likely to feel as if you "need" a sweet treat to reward yourself for all the hard work you did.

Give yourself a break. Let the mantra "progress, not perfection" be your guide, says Albers. Focus on small victories, giving yourself credit, instead of fixating on your failures. You know from running, the inner critic is a lot less motivating than a compassionate inner voice. Have the same compassion for yourself that you'd offer a good friend who was struggling with unhealthy habits. Life is about making progress each day; it's not about being perfect all the time.

Get support. Reach out to a buddy who shares or even just understands your struggle. Connect with an online or on-the-ground group that can provide support, empathy, and guidance.

Find healthy alternatives. Rather than trying to wrestle your willpower to the ground every time you have a craving, think about healthy alternatives that actually will satisfy you when you have the urge to eat. When you're feeling sad or lonely, would it help to call, write, or e-mail a friend? If you tend to eat when you're in need of distraction or relief from boredom, it might help to keep mindless magazines or books around for when you're bored. You may find relief from angry energy by playing a musical instrument. Rather than just trying to break yourself of bad habits, think about trying to grow new habits, Albers recommends. When you find a strategy for dealing with emotional discomfort that provides genuine relief, you'll be naturally inclined to stick with it.

Build an environment that supports your goals. If you've ever been on a diet or tried to stop eating a food you love—whether it's chocolate, potato chips, or cereal—you've probably discovered what scientists have now proven: If your diet feels like you're in a daily wrestling match with your willpower, it's not likely to last. Our modern world doesn't help matters. Food is everywhere. It seems you can't go to a cash register anywhere without being presented with candy to grab and go. And many fast-food restaurants offer extra-large servings of everything, often at a discount, so you're encouraged to buy them. And those environmental triggers can be just as powerful as the emotional factors that drive our eating decisions. Over the past 25 years, researcher Brian Wansink has been probing the environmental cues that cause us to overeat the wrong things. Wansink points out that even after people are made aware of cues that drive them to eat when they're not hungry, they still tend to fall back into bad habits. "Most people want to think that they're too smart to get fooled," he says. "I guess we like to think that we're a lot more smart and in control of our lives than we are. And no one likes to be told that they're wrong." In his book *Slim by Design: Mindless Eating Solutions for Everyday Life,* Wansink outlines easy steps anyone can take at home, at work, and in schools to eliminate or minimize those external cues to eat, to make living and office spaces more conducive to weight loss and active living. To minimize the mindless noshing, put the food out of sight. Make it more convenient to grab and cook healthy foods and avoid lounging around, watching TV, listening to music, or working in the kitchen.

Nikki's Story: Beating Depression-Driven Eating

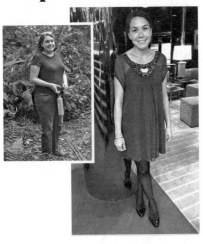

NIKKI MARSHALL had always been a size 10. But after she had her son Charlie, everything changed. She was so focused on taking care of him, she didn't have the time to think about her own nourishment. She'd shovel in dinner while standing up in the kitchen, barely even tasting her food. After exhausting days with the baby, she felt like she deserved a sweet treat, such as take-out food or a few glasses of wine. At the grocery store, she beelined for chocolate milk or a candy bar.

"Treating myself all the time was a big part of my weight gain," she says. Boredom and depression also prompted mindless eating. "I was trying to eat my feelings away!"

Two years after giving birth to her son, she felt stuck at size 16.

Getting up and down off the floor—which she constantly had to do as a preschool teacher—felt embarrassing.

Friends had dropped their baby weight quickly. "That really depressed me because I thought something was wrong with me," she says. And even though she wasn't pregnant, the worst part was, people kept asking, "When are you due?"

"I became extremely depressed and found myself using food as a way to cheer myself up, which would just make me more depressed later on," says Marshall, 38, from Melbourne, Australia. "It was a vicious cycle. I lost faith in myself and began to pull away from my family and friends."

As she got bigger, she started making excuses to avoid social events because she had no clothes that fit and felt embarrassed about her size. "Secluding myself was the worst thing I could have done, because it gave me the opportunity to sit at home and eat," she says. And it became a vicious cycle.

"The bigger I became, the more depressed I became, and the more depressed I became, the more I would eat," she says. Though she was aware on some level of what was happening, she also felt like she couldn't stop.

Marshall joined two different gyms but would quit after a few weeks, feeling embarrassed about working out in front of people at the size she was. The quitting just made her feel like a failure, which led her to eat more.

Inspired by a friend's weight loss and happy mood, she tried a couch-to-5-K program and started running. In 8 months, she lost 50 pounds. "I have energy, I sleep well, I have a positive outlook on life," she says. "I feel like me again."

Running was a key part of what got her out of her funk. In the course of the weight loss and the training, she has built up to running three times a week and has finished a 31-minute 5-K. Now she's training for her first 10-K. But the biggest reward was how it made her feel about working out. As the weight has come off, she can hold a faster pace for a longer amount of time. "When I first started running when I was heavy, I often felt as if my feet were barely shuffling along the ground," she says. "Now there is a fluidity to my running. I feel like I have a rhythm when I run."

She also started practicing habits that have been proven to work for long-term weight loss: She started eating breakfast. She made smart swaps, forgoing her usual morning latte for a cup of black tea, along with a bowl of oatmeal with blueberries and cinnamon. She started eating lots of fruits and vegetables and keeping meals regularly timed—noon for lunch and dinner by 6:30 p.m. She also started incorporating whole grains such as quinoa and brown rice. She scaled back her portions. She started planning her meals, stocking her fridge and pantry with healthy options, and made time in her schedule to prepare healthy foods. But the biggest impact came from the changes she made to why and how she ate.

She stopped eating in front of her phone, computer, and TV. "This made a huge difference," she says. "I no longer mindlessly eat and instead savor and enjoy my food." She also started to drink water and mint tea, and keeps healthy snacks around for when she feels the urge to eat but isn't hungry.

She'll also treat herself to cupcakes or fries from time to time. For her, complete deprivation is a recipe for disaster. "If I deny myself rich foods completely, I'll just want to binge on them," she says. "But I no longer see them as 'treats I deserve.' Instead, I view them as 'sometimes foods.' I have removed the stigma attached to them and no longer feel like a failure or get depressed if I eat something rich."

She credits running with helping to turn her mood around; in the first month she got a sense of accomplishment from sticking with her plan. The slow, steady increase of couch-to-5-K felt doable and gave her something to be proud of. Posting her runs on social media elicited an outpouring of support from her family and friends. That further bolstered her mood. It also helped her insomnia, which gave her energy to move more throughout the day.

She has also made big changes in the ways she copes with stress. If she needs a lift after a stressful or depressing day, she'll crank up the headphones and head out for a run instead of reaching for food.

When the old urge to eat because of stress or depression arises, she tries to distract herself with her favorite hobbies, music, errands, or by calling friends or family while she waits for the urge to pass. She has also started seeing a counselor and keeping a journal. "Letting my feelings out through talking or writing negates the urge to 'eat my feelings away,'" she says.

To keep temptation far at bay, she keeps only healthy food in the house. Though there have been slip-ups, she's focused on letting them go instead of letting them drag her down: "Instead of letting them depress me, I start fresh the next day and recommit to my healthy lifestyle."

THE TAKEAWAY

Do a gut check. The next time you reach for food, take a minute to investigate whether your urge to eat is driven by a biological signal such as a rumbling, empty stomach, or whether you're reaching for food to satisfy a deeper longing for mental or emotional comfort.

Put on the brakes. Find a way to slow down your eating so you can enjoy your food more, give your body a chance to register whether it's full, and avoid eating more calories than you need. You might try applying the 2-minute rule (waiting 2 minutes before satisfying a craving for food), sitting down before you eat, or eating with your nondominant hand.

Make a list of nonfood forms of relief. Everyone experiences stress, emotional discomfort, and mental anguish from time to time. Make a list of strategies that will genuinely provide relief from those states. List as many strategies as possible so you have lots of options for a variety of different moods or circumstances.

29

How Stress Impacts Your Weight and Your Running Life

Yes, it's stressful when you can't reach your feel-great weight or your finish-line goals. But there's pretty good evidence that chronic stress can also get in the way of your weight-loss goals.

Not only can it impact the calories you consume, it can also impact your ability to burn them. Stress can affect sleep, cause fatigue, compromise your form and endurance, and even put you at risk for injury. "All those things can have a profound effect on performance and injury risks," says Anthony Luke, a sports medicine doctor at UCSF Medical Center. "It's actually a pretty complex web."

Stress can dampen the immune system too. In a March 2013 study published in the journal *Neuroimmunomodulation*, the higher marathon trainees scored for things such as anxiety and worry 1 month before their races, the worse off their immune systems were.[1]

Some of the impact of stress is driven by behavior—e.g., reaching for chocolate when you're stressed—and some of it boils down to biochemistry. Here's what you need to know about how your state of mind can impact your waistline and your race times.

Your Body on Stress

When we're stressed, our bodies perceive an imminent threat. In response, our glands release adrenaline and cortisol so we can fight or flee (hence the so-called fight-or-flight response). Cortisol tells the body to stockpile calories to contend with that threat and to store those calories where they're most likely to stick—deep within the belly.

That's why stress can rev up your appetite for sugary, fatty comfort foods—which deliver the biggest calorie punch per ounce—and why the pounds are so problematic. Visceral belly fat, which is underneath the chest and abdominal walls, has been linked to a higher risk of diabetes and heart disease.

What's more, overexposure to cortisol can cause your muscles to break down at a faster rate than they do when you're not feeling stressed, says Shawn Talbott, a Salt Lake City nutritional biochemist who has completed more than 100 marathons and triathlons. When muscle breakdown is added to increased appetite and increased visceral belly fat, stress creates a "triple whammy" for anyone looking to lose weight through running, Talbott says.

Recent research suggests that stress seems to amplify the effects of junk food. In a study published in the April 2014 issue of *Psychoneuroendocrinology*,[2] researchers found that highly stressed people who eat a lot of fatty, sugary foods are more prone to health risks than unstressed people who eat the same food. One study suggests that when people are stressed, fat cells grow faster in response to

CHEW ON THIS

Being stressed may be worse for your race times—and your waistline—than any traditional overuse injury. In addition to derailing your sleep and sapping the energy you need to run, stress can drive you to eat and possibly even amplify the ill effects of sweet and salty foods.

junk food than when they're not stressed, says the lead author of the study, Kirstin Aschbacher, PhD, an assistant professor in the department of psychiatry at the University of California, San Francisco. This has been proven in lab animals but never in people.[3]

Here are some proven strategies you can use to stress less and protect your body—and your waistline—from its most harmful effects.

Sleep. It's been proven to lower cortisol levels.[4] Lack of sleep is "probably one of the most underappreciated stress triggers out there," says Talbott. If you're working out hard, trying to lose weight, and hitting a plateau, one of the problems may be that you're only getting 6 hours of sleep every night.

Be mindful. Research is now proving that mindfulness-based interventions for stress eating reduce both cortisol and visceral fat. A study published in the October 2011 issue of the *Journal of Obesity* found that increasing mindfulness and responsiveness to bodily sensations reduced anxiety, eating in response to external food cues, and emotional eating. In the study, those who had the greatest reduction in stress lost the most fat.[5] One component of mindfulness training involves teaching people to become aware of the cues of hunger and satiety, rather than responding to automatic eating behaviors, says Frederick Hecht, MD, a coauthor of the study and a professor of medicine at University of California, San Francisco. Another element is using mindfulness techniques to respond to stress and difficult emotions. "That may be easier to maintain than calorie counting for the rest of your life," he says. "I don't think it's going to be a magic bullet, but it is going to add to their weight-loss strategies," he says. (For more on mindful eating, see Chapter 30.)

Eat your fruits and veggies. "The more stress you're under, the more varied your phytonutrient intake should be," says Talbott. Brightly colored fruits and vegetables are not only good for you but there's also emerging evidence that they can help shield your body from damage from stress, he says. "The more you get, the more you're going to protect yourself." Talbott is working on mapping out exactly how certain phytonutrients, such as green tea extract, turmeric, and resveratrol, can shield the body from the effects of cortisol "and how they can short-circuit that stress response at a cellular level."

Jennifer's Story: **The Power of Positive Thinking**

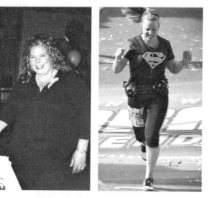

JENNIFER HITTLE has accomplished what a lot of people dream about: She shed more than half her body weight, and she has maintained her 140-pound weight for 12 years on her 5'4" frame. She went from walking around her neighborhood at night to finishing the Boston Marathon in 5:12.

But the most radical transformation actually happened on the inside. To reach those goals, she had to learn to believe in herself, even when she stumbled.

"I had to learn to stop beating myself up," she says. "That was the very thing that sabotaged my efforts."

Hittle had tried several fad diets, but every attempt just derailed her further.

"Every time I would do one of these diets and it failed, I would fill my head with so much negativity, saying, 'You'll always be fat, you'll never lose weight, why did you even try?'" she recalls.

The shame and regret would be so consuming, she'd spend up to a month drowning her sorrows in more junk food.

Then one day something clicked. "I realized the one thing I had never focused on was my thoughts," she says.

Indeed, what ultimately worked for Hittle was changing the patterns of thinking that had fostered such an unhealthy lifestyle.

From that point on if she slipped up, instead of turning to bad food she would try to work out a little longer that day. If she ate an unhealthy dinner, she made sure to start the next day with egg whites. "I could go to bed knowing that tomorrow was a new day," she says. "It wasn't always perfect, but it was a big part of my weight-loss journey."

She also had to change the negative messages she was sending herself about her weight-loss efforts.

"Every time I'd say something terrible to myself, it would keep the cycle going," she says. "I made a vow that I needed to support myself the way I would a friend or a loved one."

If she indulged in one off-the-diet brownie, she would vow to work out longer than usual the next day. "That immediately stopped the voices that would cause me to go for the whole pan," she says. And it helped with exercise too. "Before, I would say something like 'Look at you, you're so fat you can't even make it around the block. You're breathing so heavy. Why even try?!' This is something I would never say to anyone! The new me chose to say, 'Great job! You're out here walking tonight. Doesn't it feel good?' It wasn't always perfect, but I chose my self-talk very carefully. It's gotten much easier."

She learned to think like an athlete; instead of thinking about diet and exercise, she started to think of herself as a competitor who fuels and trains.

And she learned that she didn't have to be perfect.

"The scale fluctuates, and sometimes you make poor food choices," she says. "But when I believed in myself, I stopped beating myself up over it. I realized that it's the journey, not the destination."

Creating an infrastructure in her life that supports positive thinking and maintenance goals has been critical.

"There will be times the going gets tough that you will need to remember why you want it," she says.

When she needs a motivational boost, she turns to outlets such as Pinterest, YouTube, and her favorite health magazines.

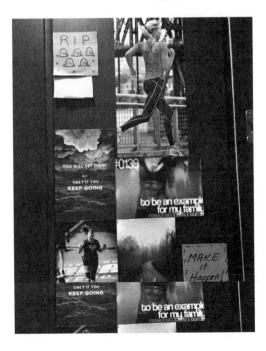

And in her kitchen she set up a vision board to remind her of her goals in key places where she might be at risk for getting off track. On the board she posts motivational pictures and notes.

"If I'm dragging my feet to get out and run, I just open the cupboard door," she says. "If my girls' goldfish crackers start looking good, I open the cupboard door."

She even made a graveyard out of sticky notes with tombstones that said "1 pound" to represent every pound she lost. If she's up a pound or two before racing season, this helps her set small goals to get back down to racing weight. "I like the visual of placing 1 pound (or sticky note) at a time in the graveyard," she says.

And it helped her face down temptation during a summer barbecue at her home, the day before a 19-mile training run. "When I was about to reach for a drink, I opened the cupboard and looked at my vision board instead," she says. "It reminded me that although I could indulge in that moment, I would rather rock my training run and celebrate in Chicago after the marathon."

THE TAKEAWAY

Stop the stress eating. Though sweet and salty foods beckon when you're stressed, times of stress are when junk food can wreak the most havoc on your waistline and your long-term health. Have a list of convenient and easy activities you can do when you're stressed to help you avoid junk food.

Get some sleep. Aim for 8 hours per night. Studies show that if you're chronically sleep deprived, you're going to be more prone to the damaging effect of stress.

Get quality meals and mileage. The compounds in fruits and veggies help reduce risk of chronic diseases that stress creates. When you're feeling stressed, reach for a variety of fruits and vegetables to get the protective benefits their phytonutrients create.

30

From Mindful to Mindless: How to Create Healthy Habits That Last for Life

Exciting as it is, the idea of embarking on a new weight-loss plan can be overwhelming. We know how much physical and emotional effort lasting change requires. If you have attempted change and stumbled in the past—and who hasn't?—even just the act of aspiring to change and risking failure can feel exhausting.

After all, most people assume that to achieve your feel-great weight, you'll have to exercise herculean feats of willpower and white-knuckle it through minefields that make healthy eating and exercise so very challenging.

Wouldn't it be great if we could just flip a switch in our brain that would force us to eat the healthiest foods in the healthiest amounts and get the most effective workouts? That may be impossible, but habits may be the next best thing.

Once you become aware of the emotional and environmental triggers between you and your goals and get some perspective on your own desires and temperament, you can use that information to create

CHEW ON THIS

Investing the time to form healthy habits can pay off when you need it most. A study in the June 2013 issue of *Journal of Personality and Social Psychology*[1] concluded that during times of high stress, when reserves of energy, willpower, and self-control feel most depleted, you'll be likely to fall back on habits, whether they're good or bad.

habits that set you up for success. By setting up a series of carefully crafted habits, you can put your healthiest eating and most effective training practices on autopilot.

Habit: A Force of Freedom

The term *habit* has an austere connotation; it implies servitude and obligation. It sounds downright unpleasant. But as Gretchen Rubin explains in her book *Better Than Before: Mastering the Habits of Our Everyday Lives,*[2] habits can actually liberate us from fretting about what to eat, when to exercise, and how to reach and maintain our feel-great weight.

"Habits are freeing and energizing," says Rubin. "They save us from the draining and difficult work of making decisions and exercising our self-control."

Indeed, if you're constantly questioning "Should I eat that?" you're bound to exhaust your emotional energy, which is a finite resource and usually depleted when we need it most, she says.

What's more, each time you practice a healthy habit, it gets stronger and more automatic, so you don't have to muster up as much willpower to do it.

"Habits make it easier. Your behavior goes on autopilot," says Rubin. "The more you do it the more you grease the wheels. You don't have to use up your decision making. You have a higher resolve. What's more, you'll have that precious resolve when you need it the most—to spend on the people and the causes you most care about. You haven't worn yourself down wondering 'Should I go to the gym today?' You could spend the whole day fussing about it and never go."

The Most Effective Habit-Making Habits

We don't mean to make habit-forming sound easy—it's not. (There's a whole canon of self-help literature on the topic for a reason.) Here are some universals about effective habit creation that Rubin learned. They can help you make your own eating and exercise life more effective than before, so you can reach your weight-loss and racing goals.

Respect yourself. This is probably the most important thing. "We can build our habits only on the foundation of our own nature," says Rubin. "You are who you are. You can be yourself." Change *is* definitely possible, but personality transplants are highly unlikely. So as you're setting up habits, do so with an honest understanding of your own nature. If you're a night owl, don't vow to start daily 5 a.m. workouts. If you have a rebellious nature, starting a diet that requires keeping a daily food diary isn't a good idea. Focus on changing the situation to suit your desires and inclinations. "That's way easier," she says. Of course, it can take some time to figure out what those desires and inclinations are. "Often people aren't even aware of what they are or haven't thought about it," Rubin says. An important part of this is understanding how you tend to respond to inner and outer expectations, and whether you fall into one of four categories that Rubin outlines. Are you an upholder who responds readily to both outer and inner expectations? Are you a questioner who challenges all expectations—unless you think they're justified? Are you an obliger who can easily meet someone else's expectations but not your own? Or are you a rebel who resists all expectations, whether they're internal or come from someone else? Knowing and embracing your own nature will help you frame your habits in a way that is most helpful to you, so you're most likely to follow them.

Show a little compassion. "A lot of people think that if they load themselves with guilt and shame, they'll energize themselves," says Rubin. "Research shows just the opposite." Usually people feel so bad about themselves, they turn to the very bad habit that got them into trouble. Show a little compassion—don't say anything to yourself that you wouldn't tell a good friend—and you'll get the energy to engage and try again. Don't try to pretend you're someone you're not, she counsels.

Convenience matters. If you've ever attempted to drown your sorrows in a pint of ice cream, you know: "Often with a bad habit, you're in the middle of it before you even notice it," says Rubin. That's why it's so important to make anything you don't want to do inconvenient, and anything you do want to do as easy as possible. "We are extremely influenced by convenience and inconvenience," she says. So if you don't want to indulge in cookies, don't buy them. You'll have to get dressed and leave the house to go get them, which will discourage you from doing so. If you want to avoid eating the entire family-size bag of potato chips, get single-serving bags. That way you'll have to think about opening a second package if you want to eat more than one serving. Just having to open that second package will interrupt the momentum of eating enough to make you stop in your tracks.

Treat yourself. Have a list of tasks that feel like treats for you and make sure they don't have anything to do with eating, drinking, or exercise. Treats are a critical part of life. "When we give ourselves treats, we feel recharged and taken care of," says Rubin. "You have to give yourself a lot of healthy treats so that you don't feel deprived and depleted." Trouble occurs, however, because the most popular forms of treats involve eating and drinking. When we're feeling low and in need of a lift, food is often our first thought. And it's no wonder. It's legal, and the cheapest and most convenient form of aesthetic pleasure there is. In our culture, we're conditioned to think of foods as treats. What's more, many adults don't have a lot of stress-relieving treats that don't involve food. Make a list of things you can use anytime you're feeling low and need a pick-me-up. Maybe it's a podcast, new music, a new book, a video, a manicure, or an hour to wander through the camping store to ogle the gear. Rubin discovered that for a lot of people it's ironing. "Do whatever works for you," she says. "Just don't use food."

No man is an island. "We're enormously influenced by other people's habits," Rubin says. "If you want to form a particular habit, think carefully about what people around you are doing." If they're doing a good job, that's helpful. If they're not, or they're actively sabotaging your goals, plan how you're going to contend with them. Think about the frenemies who tell you one cupcake won't hurt that diet, or the food-pushers at family meals who tell you you're obsessed because you're not going to indulge in brisket. Or what about the partner who gives you grief for getting up for that Saturday morning run? You can have an iron will, but you can't be immune to other people around you.

Erin's Story: How Convenience Became Key to Running and Weight-Loss Success

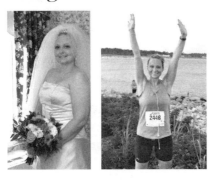

ERIN MULLANE hit her get-up-or-give-up moment on her daughter's first birthday, in 2013.

"I was overweight, tired, and sitting on the sidelines of life," says Mullane. Though she couldn't run for a full minute, she signed up for a 5-K five months away, downloaded a couch-to-5-K app, and committed to running three times a week.

Since then, she has lost 65 pounds and has kept it off. She has finished three half-marathons and many shorter races. Though running played a leading role in her success, some of the most powerful changes she made happened off the road.

She ate more vegetables, swapped soda for water, dropped butter and salt, shrank bread and pasta servings, and started cooking more often than dining out. Pizza, fast food, and potato chips went by the wayside.

And the 36-year-old found out what a lot of people do: Keeping the weight off was an even bigger challenge than losing it in the first place. "Maintaining my weight loss has not been easy," says Mullane, a speech-language pathologist from New London, Connecticut. "It's so easy to get back into old habits."

Though she was working out a lot, she was rewarding her efforts with extra calories that ultimately showed up on the scale. She spent time wondering, "How much do I actually burn on a 9-mile run?" and "Can I have that cupcake if I ran 3 miles? Five miles?"

She ended up joining Weight Watchers just to maintain her weight, as it helped her keep track of her calorie consumption and burn to get the balance right.

What's worked for her? A just-one-bite rule for sweets. She doesn't deprive herself of anything. But she takes one bite, then walks away. "Once a minute or two has passed, that one bite becomes just that," says Mullane. "A satisfying taste of something delicious. If you allow that second, third, fourth bite, you are less satisfied. Because you might feel more guilty."

Taking control of her food environment has been key. When she's headed out to book club, she takes a healthy dish so she'll have at least one option.

When friends want to get together, she suggests meeting for a run or a walk instead of lunch. When going out to dinner, she'll pick the restaurant and preview menus online so she can decide what she'll order before she gets there.

She no longer stops for fast food. And she's not afraid to splurge on healthier, but often more expensive, higher-quality cuts of meat, individually wrapped snacks, or precut fruit to save time.

"I save money by not going out to eat much," she says. "Spending a little extra at the grocery store is totally worth it!"

THE TAKEAWAY

Know yourself. As you're making a list of healthy habits you'd like to adopt, think about your tendencies and desires and make sure they fit within that framework.

Make a list of nonfood rewards. Make a list of pick-me-ups: walk your dog, call a friend, give yourself 30 minutes of Googling with abandon. Play the piano. Clean out a drawer. Brush your teeth. Take a shower. Look at photos from your recent vacation. Do whatever gives you relief when you feel low. Write this list down and keep it in a place where you can see it.

Surround yourself with support. Connect with other people who are working on weight loss and exercise or struggling with the same unique obstacles. If it's not convenient to meet them in person, connect with them online on a regular basis. That will make you feel less self-conscious about your efforts and get support you need to stay on track.

ACKNOWLEDGMENTS

We would like to sincerely thank all the experts who so generously shared their time and expertise for this book. They include Amby Burfoot, Kim Larson, Jenny Hadfield, Janet Hamilton, Jenna Bell, Susan Paul, Steve Hertzler, Ted Spiker, Blake Russell, Richard Hecht, Brian Wansink, Susan Albers, Gretchen Rubin, Riley Nickols, Dee McCaffrey, and Shawn Talbott. Thank you to Mark Weinstein, David Willey, and John Atwood for believing in the project and making it a reality.

We are very grateful to all the runners who so bravely shared their personal stories about shrinking their waistlines and their race times in the hopes of encouraging, supporting, and guiding others. Without your courage and candor, we would not have been able to write this book.

We owe the biggest thanks to our families. We simply cannot say loudly or often enough just how much we appreciate our husbands—Peter Van Allen and Jason Bede. Thank you for taking such good care of our sons, our chores, and us during the many months of typing. We would not have been able to do this without you. Finally, thank you to our sons—Noah Van Allen and Miller and Hunter Bede. You were so patient and forgiving while your mommies wrote this book. We're looking forward to lots of long walks, afternoons in the park, games of pirate, and rounds of fort-building; we've missed it all as much as you have.

MEAL PLANS

1,600-CALORIE MEAL PLAN

BREAKFAST

³/₄ cup bran flakes cereal

6 ounces light (reduced-calorie) low-fat yogurt

8 medium strawberries

8–16 ounces water

MORNING SNACK

1 cup low-fat (1%) cottage cheese

1 medium apple

8–16 ounces water

LUNCH

Chopped chicken salad made from:

2 cups spring mix

¹/₄ cup each chopped green and red bell pepper

¹/₂ cup chopped tomato

2 ounces goat cheese

³/₄ cup chopped grilled chicken

2 tablespoons reduced-fat balsamic dressing

1 whole grain dinner roll

8–16 ounces water

AFTERNOON SNACK

2 graham cracker squares topped with 1 tablespoon
natural peanut butter and 1 medium banana

8–16 ounces water

DINNER

Pan-seared salmon with garlic and asparagus over rice:

In a nonstick skillet, heat 1 tablespoon canola oil. Once oil is hot, add 1 clove
garlic and 6 chopped asparagus spears and sauté for 1 to 2 minutes. Add
3 ounces Atlantic salmon and cook until fish pulls apart easily with a fork.
Serve atop 1 cup cooked brown, long-grain rice.

8–16 ounces water

Approximate Daily Intake

Calories: 1,578; Total fat: 45 g; Saturated fat: 9 g; Trans fat: 0 g;
Carbohydrate: 194 g; Protein: 99 g; Fiber: 27 g

2,000-CALORIE MEAL PLAN

BREAKFAST

$^1/_2$ cup old-fashioned oats made with 8 ounces fat-free milk

1 medium apple

8 ounces green tea with sliced lemon

8 ounces water

MORNING SNACK

$^1/_4$ cup hummus

$^1/_2$ whole grain pita, toasted

1 cup baby carrots

8–16 ounces water

LUNCH

1 turkey sandwich with 2 slices whole wheat bread
and 2 ounces low-sodium sliced turkey

1 cup chopped romaine lettuce topped with
2 tablespoons low-fat vinaigrette

1 cup fat-free vanilla Greek yogurt

8–16 ounces water

AFTERNOON SNACK

$1^1/_4$ cups high-fiber, high-protein cereal

1 medium banana

8 ounces fat-free milk

8 ounces green tea with sliced lemon

DINNER

3 ounces baked salmon

1 cup brown rice

1 cup steamed broccoli

8–16 ounces water

EVENING SNACK

1 ounce Cheddar cheese

6 whole wheat crackers

$^1/_2$ cup sliced cucumber

Approximate Daily Intake

Calories: 1,990; Total fat: 44 g; Saturated fat: 26 g; Trans fat: 0 g;
Carbohydrate: 292 g; Protein: 108 g; Fiber: 46 g

2,500-CALORIE MEAL PLAN

BREAKFAST

1 scrambled egg

1 cup cooked spinach

2 slices whole wheat bread

1 ounce Cheddar cheese

8 ounces green tea

8 ounces water with lemon

MORNING SNACK

1 ounce (49 kernels) dry-roasted pistachios

1 cup fresh mixed berries

8–16 ounces water

LUNCH

Salad with 2 cups shredded romaine lettuce, 2 tablespoons
low-fat vinaigrette, $\frac{1}{2}$ cup canned chickpeas

1 cup couscous

1 whole wheat dinner roll

3 ounces grilled chicken breast

8–16 ounces water with lemon

AFTERNOON SNACK

Smoothie made by blending 2 scoops 100% whey protein powder
(chocolate), 1 medium banana, 8 ounces fat-free milk, and 1 cup ice

DINNER

3 ounces roasted pork tenderloin

$\frac{1}{2}$ cup baked sweet potato

1 cup cooked broccoli

1 whole wheat dinner roll

1 tablespoon butter

8–16 ounces water

EVENING SNACK

1 tablespoon peanut butter

1 large apple

8–16 ounces water

Approximate Daily Intake

Calories: 2,550; Total fat: 84 g; Saturated fat: 20 g; Trans fat: 0 g;
Carbohydrate 288 g; Protein: 158 g; Fiber: 58 g

3,000-CALORIE MEAL PLAN

BREAKFAST

5.3 ounces low-fat fruited Greek yogurt

1 cup fresh blueberries

³/₄ cup granola

Coffee or tea as desired

MORNING SNACK

1 smoothie made with 2 scoops 100% whey protein powder,
1 cup baby spinach, 1 cup frozen blueberries, 1 cup fat-free milk

LUNCH

Burrito bowl: 1 cup brown rice, ¹/₂ cup low-sodium black beans,
1 cup corn, ¹/₄ cup salsa, 6 ounces grilled chicken

1 cup cooked broccoli

1 medium stone fruit

8–16 ounces water

AFTERNOON SNACK

1 rice cake

1 tablespoon almond butter

8–16 ounces water with lemon

DINNER

Spaghetti and meatballs: 1¹/₂ cups whole wheat pasta,
1 cup Italian-style tomato sauce, and 4 ounces meatballs

1 cup green beans

1 ounce Monterey Jack cheese

8–16 ounces water

EVENING SNACK

1 ounce roasted unsalted almonds

¹/₄ cup dried cranberries

8–16 ounces water

Approximate Daily Intake

Calories: 3,040; Total fat: 80 g; Saturated fat: 21 g; Trans fat: 0 g;
Carbohydrate: 400 g; Protein: 180 g; Fiber: 62 g

RUN TO LOSE RULES OF THUMB

Best balance of carbs, protein, and fats. To fuel your running, at least 55 percent of your daily calories should come from wholesome carbohydrates (such as whole grains, fresh fruits, and vegetables), and the balance of your calories should come from lean proteins and healthy fats. (See page 39 for more.)

Pack in the Protein. Aim for 0.55 to 0.9 gram of protein per pound of body weight per day to recover from workouts and continue to build strength and fitness. The more miles you're logging and the more strength training you're doing, the more protein you're likely to need. So if you weigh 130 pounds, target 72 to 117 grams per day. A 195-pound runner will need to aim for approximately 107 to 175 grams per day.

Get your fiber. To boost heart health and keep the GI tract running efficiently, have plenty of fiber each day. The American Heart Association recommends that men should aim for 38 grams of fiber per day and women should target 25 grams of fiber per day. (See page 122 for more.)

Stay hydrated every day. To avoid dehydration, which can drag down your running performance, you'll want to fill up on calorie-free fluids until your urine runs a light lemonade or straw color. Many experts recommend you start with a goal of consuming approximately half your body weight in ounces of fluids per day. So if you weigh 200 pounds, try to consume at least 100 ounces of calorie-free fluids each day. If you weigh 140 pounds, aim for 70 ounces of fluids per day. Sip fluids throughout the day so you're not chugging huge amounts just before your run. (See page 94 for more.)

Steer clear of sugar. To keep your sugar intake low, aim for less than 10 grams of sugar per serving. Look at the ingredient list; if sugar is one of the first three ingredients, choose another product. (See page 62 for more.)

Choose the right sports food at the right time. Whole foods are always the best choice. But when whole foods are out of reach or your stomach simply doesn't tolerate them before a workout, a sports bar, shake, or other engineered food can meet your needs. Whether you're choosing whole foods or sports foods, here's what to look for.

- **Prerun snack:** For a run of 60 minutes or less at an easy effort, limit it to 200 calories or less, with less than 10 grams of fat and 7 grams of fiber.

- **Midrun refueling:** If you're going to be on a run for 1, 2, or 3 hours at a time, you want to aim for a product that's going to provide 30 to 60 grams of carbs per hour you're on the road.

- **Postrun refueling:** After a speed session or a long run, have a protein shake, smoothie, sports bar, or snack with a 2:1 ratio of carbs to protein to help you bounce back strong. For more, see Chapter 22.

- **Meal replacement:** Make sure the bar or shake doesn't contain more calories than you'd have in a regular meal. Look at the serving size; some items have more than one serving per pack.

Race day nutrition (for 5-Ks and 10-Ks): Consume foods that are low in fat, fiber, and protein. For each nutrient, aim for under 10 grams per serving unless you are sensitive to fiber and, in that case, limit to 7 grams or less. (See page 178 for more.)

- Keep your prerace snack under 200 calories; make sure it's rich in carbs.

- Drink 20 ounces of fluids 2 to 3 hours before the race.

- Drink 10 ounces of fluids in the 20 minutes before the race.

When to carb-load: Carb-loading for a full marathon is the best way to increase the chances of running your best race. Carb-loading for a half-marathon is only marginally necessary. For any race of less than 90 minutes, carb-loading is totally unnecessary, and chances are good that it may actually hurt your chances of running well on race day. (See page 181 for more.)

Calculated carb-load: See page 183 for more.

Marathons

7 days before the race: Consume 2.3 grams of carbs per pound of body weight each day.

1 to 3 days before the race: Consume 3.6 to 5.5 grams of carbs per pound of body weight each day.

Half-Marathons

1 to 3 days before the race: Consume 2.5 to 4 grams of carbs per pound of body weight each day.

Refueling on the road: For any run of 75 minutes or more, refuel while you're on the road. Consume 30 to 60 grams of carbs per hour. Consume them from the time you start your run, *before* you become hungry or starved for energy. Refuel at regular intervals throughout the run—say every 15 to 30 minutes—to keep your energy levels stable. (See page 190 for more.)

Avoid unwanted pit stops on the run. To avoid GI distress, keep your prerun meal or snack to these per-serving limits.

- Less than 7 grams of fiber
- Less than 10 grams of fat
- Less than 10 grams of protein

The longer you go, the more you'll need to refuel. The longer you'll be on the road, the more carbs you should consume each hour. If you're heading out for a 75-minute run, try 30 grams of carbs per hour. If you're heading out for 150 minutes, aim closer to 60 grams of carbs per hour. For runs that last longer than 3 hours, aim for 90 grams of carbs per hour. (See page 191 for more.)

Refueling with sports drinks: If you're using sports drinks to refuel while you're on the road, stick with drinks that have less than 14 to 17 grams of carbs per 8 ounces. Runners with sensitive stomachs should aim for the lower end of this range or even less. For best tolerance, look for drinks with multiple sources of carbs—such as glucose, fructose, sucrose, or maltodextrin—which your body will absorb better than a single source by itself. (See page 193 for more.)

Fueling up with whole foods: When you're using whole foods to refuel on the road, stick with foods that are low in fat, fiber, and protein. Look for foods with less than 3 to 5 grams per serving. Start there and see how you feel. Depending on how tough your gut is, you may be able to tolerate more. (See page 194 for more.)

Refueling Postworkout: Research has proven that carbs and protein are the most effective nutrients for helping the body recover after a workout. The carbs in your recovery meal restock your spent glycogen stores. Aim for approximately 0.5 gram of carbohydrate per pound of body weight. So if you weigh 150 pounds, have a recovery meal with 75 grams of carbs. Adding a small amount of protein to a recovery meal will speed your muscle repair and recovery. Aim for at least 15 to 25 grams of protein in your recovery meal. (See page 200 for more.)

Rehydrating postworkout: How do you know if you're properly rehydrated after a tough workout? Do the sweat test. Weigh yourself naked before a run, then again afterward, and determine how many ounces you lost through sweat. (Remember, 1 pound equals approximately 16 ounces.) Drink that many ounces of fluid (drink 24 ounces for each pound lost if you have another workout looming within 24 hours and need to rehydrate quickly). If you don't have access to a scale, you can simply drink until your thirst diminishes and your urine runs a light straw color. (See page 200 for more.)

Returning to Running after a Layoff

(See page 226 for more.)

IF YOU'RE OFF . . .	START RIGHT HERE
1 week or less	Pick up your plan where you left off
Up to 10 days	Start running 70% of previous mileage
15 to 30 days	Start running 60% of previous mileage
30 days to 3 months	Start running 50% of previous mileage
3 months	Start from scratch

FOOD LABEL QUICK-REFERENCE GUIDE

Reading food labels is a healthy habit that has been linked to long-term weight loss.[1] If you're not cooking them yourself, it's the only way to guarantee that you're consuming the foods with the most nutrition and the least waist-expanding additives you don't need.

Daunting as it may feel at first, once you start reading labels regularly, it becomes second nature. And you don't have to spend hours examining packaged foods before you buy them. Here's a quick guide to decoding food labels. Photocopy it and take it with you next time you go to buy food. You may be surprised by what you learn along the way!

Here are some of the most common claims seen on food packages and what they mean.[2]

Low calorie: 40 calories or less per serving

Low cholesterol: 20 milligrams or less and 2 grams or less of saturated fat per serving

Reduced: At least 25 percent less of the specified nutrient or calories than the usual product. This doesn't necessarily mean a product is "low calorie," "low fat," or even a healthy choice.

High in/rich in/excellent source of: Provides 20 percent or more of the Daily Value of a specified nutrient per serving

Good source of: Provides 10 to 19 percent of the Daily Value of a particular vitamin or nutrient per serving

Calorie-free: Less than 5 calories per serving

Fat-free/sugar-free: Less than 0.5 gram of fat or sugar per serving

Low fat: Less than 3 grams of fat per serving

Low carb/low sugar: At this time, these label claims are not defined.

Low sodium: 140 milligrams or less of sodium per serving

Sodium-free or salt-free: Less than 5 milligrams of sodium per serving[3]

Unsalted or no salt added: No salt has been added, but this doesn't mean the product is naturally low in total sodium.

Very low in sodium: Provides 35 milligrams or less of sodium per serving

Low in sodium or "contains a small amount of sodium": Contains 140 milligrams or less of sodium per serving

Reduced sodium or less sodium: Provides at least 25 percent less sodium than the traditional product

Percent Daily Value: The percent Daily Value (%DV) tells you how much a nutrient in a serving of food contributes to your daily diet. Two thousand calories a day is used as a reference. Your needs may be higher or lower depending on your calorie and fitness requirements.

KITCHEN ESSENTIALS

When you make your own meals, you'll be able to take the reins and more effectively achieve your weight-loss and racing goals. Yes, cooking at home is more time-consuming than pulling up to a drive-thru or picking up a packaged bar. But it doesn't have to consume your life. And it doesn't have to cost an arm and a leg. You probably already own basics, like spatulas, vegetable peelers, can openers, and whisks, but here's a list of other essentials that can help you make healthy food fast.

BASIC KITCHEN TOOLS

TOOL	FUNCTION
Salad spinner	Centrifuge-type bowl that allows you to rinse, spin, and store your lettuce (or other salad ingredients). When you get home from the grocery store, wash, chop, and spin your salad ingredients. Store the leftovers in the spinner so you always have salad on hand.
Cutting board	Save your countertops and your palms by chopping and slicing your produce, meat, and other items on a cutting board. Look for one that's lightweight and sturdy. You might choose a plastic board that's dishwasher safe. If you're looking for a natural material, bamboo is a good choice.
Nonstick skillet	While some home cooks shy away from Teflon coatings, when you're looking to cut calories and fat, a nonstick surface is your friend. Nonstick skillets allow you to "pan fry" your items without using any oil or butter.
Kitchen knives	It's difficult to prepare any dish without a good set of cutlery. And while you might be hesitant to invest in a new set, if your knives are old and dull, you risk cutting yourself as you put more effort into cutting. The most basic set should include chef's, paring, serrated, and slicing knives.
Immersion blender	Sometimes referred to as a stick blender, this is a handheld electric blender that purees food in the container in which it's being prepared (saving you the hassle of transferring your soup or smoothie ingredients from bowl to blender/food processor and back again). It can be useful for soups.
Measuring cups and spoons	These tools are essential when measuring ingredients for cooking and baking. Use them to double-check portion sizes—when you first try a new food and then a few weeks later. You might notice that your portion sizes grow over time. Measuring cups and spoons can help keep you honest and keep your waistline in check. Consider buying a few sets and keeping the correct portion inside the containers of foods you use often—like cereals, pasta, and snacks that are easy to consume.
Food scale	Use a food scale to accurately measure portions when cooking or baking (to make sure the recipe turns out as intended) or use it to stick to the proper proportions of a diet or meal plan. You can use a food scale to measure out a proper serving size instead of measuring cups and spoons (check a food's Nutrition Facts panel for the gram-weight serving size).

TOOL	FUNCTION
Recipe prep bowls/ ramekins	These tiny bowls are helpful when lining up ingredients prior to mixing. They can also be used for portion control of snacks and indulgent items. If using for portion control, check the serving size of the item and divvy only 1 serving into the ramekin. Once it's empty, you're done snacking.
Food storage containers	Choose containers that are dishwasher safe, durable, airtight, and clear. Also buy some masking tape so you can clearly mark what's in the container and the date it was made. Most leftovers should be consumed within a few days for safety reasons. If you date the item, there will be no more debating how old it is.
KITCHEN WISH LIST: KITCHEN TOOLS THAT ARE OPTIONAL BUT NOT ESSENTIAL	
Meat pounder	A meat pounder is handy for tenderizing meat (like pork loin, chicken breast, and low-fat beef, which can be tough). It also makes meat cook faster and spread out. A 3-oz portion, when pounded flat, looks a lot bigger than a deck of cards. And since you'll need to cut more pieces and take more bites, you'll be forced to eat a bit slower too.
Mandoline/ julienne slicer	A mandoline is the perfect tool if you're looking to cut veggies quickly and make them attractive. Many have straight and wavy blades that can be set to different thicknesses to create cucumber slices, carrot chips, matchstick-size zucchini slices, and more. Most also include a julienne blade that churns out carrot sticks. Look for one that has safety features like a handle that keeps your hands out of the way of the blades and blades that can be removed and easily washed.
Silicone brushes	These are handy for basting foods. Instead of drowning a food in sauce or coating a pan with copious amounts of oil, use a silicone food brush (which is heat resistant, durable, and doesn't capture quite as much sauce as natural bristle brushes) to spread just enough oil and sauce on foods as you cook. You'll save calories and ingredients.
Strainer/ colander	These make it easy to clean fruits and veggies, especially harder-to-clean items like berries. This makes it easy to keep fresh produce on hand for healthy snacking.
Fat separator	This device looks like a liquid measuring cup or pitcher but has a spout at the bottom of the cup and a strainer at the top to catch solids. Since fat naturally rises to the top of items like gravy, soup, and broth when the liquid cools, you can pour out the liquid you want to keep, and leave the artery-clogging fat behind. To use one, simply transfer the sauce or broth from the stockpot it's been cooking in, letting it cool it in the fat separator. Once the fat rises to the top, pour off the liquid you want to keep, discarding the rest. To accelerate the process, put the sauce in the fridge, allow the fat to harden, then pour off (and keep) the lower-calorie sauce, broth, or soup.
Meat thermometer	A meat thermometer lets you know if poultry, beef, or other meat items have been cooked long enough that they're safe to eat and avoid overcooking them until they're dry and tough.

RECOMMENDED READING

Here are some books where you can read more about the topics we've touched on.

The Science of Skinny by Dee McCaffrey

50 Ways to Soothe Yourself without Food by Susan Albers

Eating Mindfully by Susan Albers

Quit Comfort Eating by Susan Albers

Slim by Design by Brian Wansink

Mindless Eating by Brian Wansink

The Power of Habit by Charles Duhigg

Do Life by Ben Davis

Down Size by Ted Spiker

Eat This, Not That by David Zinczenko and Matt Goulding

Better Than Before by Gretchen Rubin

The Happiness Project by Gretchen Rubin

Move a Little, Lose a Lot by James A. Levine and Selene Yeager

Food Rules by Michael Pollan

The Complete America's Test Kitchen TV Show Cookbook 2001–2015
    by the editors of America's Test Kitchen

How to Cook Everything by Mark Bittman

The Complete Book of Food Counts
    (6th edition) by Corinne T. Netzer

The Runner's World Cookbook by Joanna Sayago Golub (ed.)

ENDNOTES

Introduction

1 gallup.com/poll/21859/close-americans-want-lose-weight.aspx.

2 M. A. Kennedy et al., "Impact of Marathon Training on Body Weight in Recreational Runners," *Medicine and Science in Sports and Exercise* 42, no. 5 (2010): S441.

3 A. Sedeaud et al., "BMI, A Performance Parameter for Speed Improvement," *PLOS ONE* 9, no. 2 (2014): e90183.

Your Run to Lose Ground Rules

1 Jack Hollis et al., "Weight Loss during the Intensive Intervention Phase of the Weight-Loss Maintenance Trial," *American Journal of Preventive Medicine* 35, no. 2 (August 2008): 118–26.

2 Ellen Van Kleef, Mitsuru Shimizu, and Brian Wansink, "Just a Bite: Considerably Smaller Snack Portions Satisfy Delayed Hunger and Craving," *Journal of Food Quality and Preference* 27, no. 1 (2013): 96–100.

3 Liisa Tyrväinena et al., "The Influence of Urban Green Environments on Stress Relief Measures: A Field Experiment," *Journal of Environmental Psychology* 38 (June 2014): 1–9.

4 R. Kumar et al., "Teammates and Social Influence Affect Weight Loss Outcomes in a Team-Based Weight Loss Competition," *Obesity* 20, no. 7 (July 2012): 1413–18.

5 Claire E. Adams and Mark R. Leary, "Promoting Self-Compassionate Attitudes toward Eating among Restrictive and Guilty Eaters," *Journal of Social and Clinical Psychology* 26, no. 10 (2007): 1120–44.

Measuring Success

1 nwcr.ws/Research/default.htm.

2 Jason P. Block et al., "Consumers' Estimation of Calorie Content at Fast Food Restaurants: Cross Sectional Observational Study," *BMJ* 2013;346:f2907.

Chapter 1: All about Carbs

1 USDA Nutrient Analysis Library: ndb.nal.usda.gov/ndb/foods/show/5735?f-gcd=&manu=&lfacet=&format=&count=&max=35&offset=&sort=&qlookup-blueberry+muffin.

2 D. J. Casa et al., "Influence of Hydration on Physiological Function and Performance during Trail Running in the Heat," *Journal of Athletic Training* 45, no. 2 (March–April 2010): 147–56.

Chapter 2: Fruits and Veggies: The Forlorn Fuel

1 nutritiondata.self.com/facts/baked-products/4818/2.

2 Heiner Boeing et al., "Critical Review: Vegetables and Fruit in the Prevention of Chronic Diseases," *European Journal of Nutrition* 51, no. 6 (2012): 637–63. PMC. Web. July 26, 2015.

3 Jennifer Di Noia, "Defining Powerhouse Fruits and Vegetables: A Nutrient Density Approach," *Preventing Chronic Disease* 11, 2014.

4 preventcancer.aicr.org/site/News2?page=NewsArticle&id=15485&news_iv _ctrl=2303.

Chapter 3: Good Grains

1 archinte.jamanetwork.com/article.aspx?articleid=2087877.

2 ncbi.nlm.nih.gov/pubmed/18175740.

3 wholegrainscouncil.org/whole-grains-101/gluten-free-whole-grains.

Chapter 4: Getting Smart about Sugar

1 2015 U.S. Dietary Guidelines, health.gov/dietaryguidelines/2015-scientific -report/PDFs/Appendix-E-2.45.pdf.

2 R. H. Lustig, L. A. Schmidt, and C. D. Brindis, "Public Health: The Toxic Truth about Sugar," *Nature* 482, no. 7383 (February 1, 2012): 27–29. doi: 10.1038/482027a.

3 S. H. Ahmed, K. Guillem, and Y. Vandaele, "Sugar Addiction: Pushing the Drug-Sugar Analogy to the Limit," *Current Opinion in Clinical Nutrition and Metabolic Care* 16, no. 4 (July 2013): 434–39.

Chapter 5: The Glycemic Index

1 John P. Kirwan et al., "Effects of Moderate and High Glycemic Index Meals on Metabolism and Exercise Performance," *Metabolism* 50, no. 7 (July 2001): 849–55.

2 M. Kern, C. J. Heslin, and R. S. Rezende. "Metabolic and performance effects of raisins versus sports gels pre-exercise feedings in cyclists." *Journal of Strength and Conditioning Research* 2007 Nov; 21(4) 1204–7.

3 glycemicindex.com.

4 F. S. Atkinson, K. Faster-Powell, and J. C. Brand Miller. "International Tables of Glycemic Index and Glycemic Load Values: 2008." *Diabetes Care.* 2008; 31(12): 2281–83.

Chapter 6: Why Fats Matter

1 gallup.com/poll/166082/americans-desire-shed-pounds-outweighs-effort.aspx.

2 K. E. Gerlach et al., "Fat Intake and Injury in Female Runners," *Journal of the International Society of Sports Nutrition* 3, no. 5 (January 2008): 1.

3 J. A. Paniagua et al., "Monounsaturated Fat-Rich Diet Prevents Central Body Fat Distribution and Decreases Postprandial Adiponectin Expression Induced by a Carbohydrate-Rich Diet in Insulin-Resistant Subjects," *Diabetes Care* 30, no. 7 (July 2007): 1717–23. Epub March 23, 2007.

4 R. Chowdhury et al., "Association of Dietary, Circulating, and Supplement Fatty Acids with Coronary Risk: A Systematic Review and Meta-analysis," *Annals of Internal Medicine* 160 (2014): 398–406.

5 fda.gov/NewsEvents/Newsroom/PressAnnouncements/ucm373939.htm.

Chapter 7: Protein

1 S. M. Pasiakos et al., "Effects of High-Protein Diets on Fat-Free Mass and Muscle Protein Synthesis Following Weight Loss: A Randomized Controlled Trial," *FASEB Journal* 27, no. 9 (2013): 3837–47.

2 Heather Leidy, Laura Ortinau, and Tia Rains, "Acute Effects of Higher Protein, Sausage and Egg-Based Convenience Breakfast Meals on Postprandial Glucose Homeostasis in Healthy, Premenopausal Women," *FASEB Journal* 28, no. 1 (April 2014, Supplement 381: 6).

3 marathonbars.com/products.php.

4 USDA Nutrient Analysis United States Department of Agriculture Agricultural Research Service, National Nutrient Database for Standard Reference Release 27. ndb.nal.usda.gov/.

Chapter 8: What to Drink

1 Douglas J. Casa et al., "Influence of Hydration on Physiological Function and Performance during Trail Running in the Heat," *Journal of Athletic Training* 45, no. 2 (2010): 147–56.

2 American College of Sports Medicine, Current Comment, "Dehydration," acsm.org/docs/current-comments/dehydrationandaging.pdf?sfvrsn=6.

3 Tamara Hew-Butler et al., "Updated Fluid Recommendation: Position Statement from the International Marathon Medical Directors Association," *Clinical Journal of Sports Medicine* 16, no. 4 (July 2006): 283–92.

4 Sophie C. Killer, Andrew K. Blannin, and Asker E. Jeukendrup, "No Evidence of Dehydration with Moderate Daily Coffee Intake: A Counterbalanced Cross-Over Study in a Free-Living Population," *PLOS ONE* (January 9, 2014).

5 American College of Sports Medicine, Current Comment, "Caffeine and Exercise Performance," acsm.org/docs/current-comments/caffeineandexercise.pdf.

6 Michel Lucas et al., "Coffee, Caffeine, and Risk of Depression among Women," *Archives of Internal Medicine* 171, no. 17 (September 26, 2011): 1571–78.

7 Ming Ding et al., "Long-Term Coffee Consumption and Risk of Cardiovascular Disease: A Systematic Review and a Dose-Response Meta-Analysis of Prospective Cohort Studies," *Circulation* 129 (2014): 643–59.

8 Shilpa N. Bhupathiraju et al., "Changes in Coffee Intake and Subsequent Risk of Type 2 Diabetes: Three Large Cohorts of US Men and Women," *Diabetologia* 57, no. 7 (July 2014): 1346–54.

9 Rachael C. Gliottoni et al.,"Effect of Caffeine on Quadriceps Muscle Pain During Acute Cycling Exercise in Low Versus High Caffeine Consumers," *International Journal of Sport Nutrition and Exercise Metabolism* 19 (2009): 150–61.

Chapter 9: Alcohol

1 US Department of Agriculture and US Department of Health and Human Services "Dietary Guidelines for Americans, 2010," PDF-2.89 MB, 7th edition (2010): Washington, DC: US Government Printing Office.

2 Richard D. Semba et al., "Resveratrol Levels and All-Cause Mortality in Older Community-Dwelling Adults," *JAMA Internal Medicine* 174, no. 7 (2014): 1077–84.

3 M. Manore, "Effect of Physical Activity on Thiamine, Riboflavin, and Vitamin B_6 Requirements," *American Journal of Clinical Nutrition* 72 (suppl) (2000): 598S–606S.

4 E. B. Parr et al., "Alcohol Ingestion Impairs Maximal Post-Exercise Rates of Myofibrillar Protein Synthesis Following a Single Bout of Concurrent Training," *PLOS ONE* 9, no. 2 (2014).

Chapter 10: Sports Foods

1 Kelly Bastone, "Raising the Bar," *Runner's World* (October 2012): 33–34.

2 diabetes.org/food-and-fitness/food/what-can-i-eat/understanding -carbohydrates/sugar-alcohols.html#sthash.SCnzeoCC.dpuf.

Chapter 11: Artificial Sweeteners

1   cancer.gov/cancertopics/causes-prevention/risk/diet/artificial-sweeteners -fact-sheet.

2   Brian Wansink and Pierre Chandon, "Can 'Low-Fat' Nutrition Labels Lead to Obesity?" *Journal of Marketing Research* 43, no. 4 (November 2006): 605–17.

3   Qing Yang, "Gain Weight by 'Going Diet'? Artificial Sweeteners and the Neurobiology of Sugar Cravings," *Yale Journal of Biology and Medicine* (June 2010): 101–8.

4   Sharon P.G. Fowler, Ken Williams, and Helen P. Hazuda., "Diet Soda Intake Is Associated with Long-Term Increases in Waist Circumference in a Biethnic Cohort of Older Adults: The San Antonio Longitudinal Study of Aging," *Journal of the American Geriatrics Society* 63, no. 4 (April 2015): 708–15.

Chapter 12: Decoding Food Labels

1   Bidisha Mandal, "Use of Food Labels as a Weight-Loss Behavior," *Journal of Consumer Affairs* 44, no. 3 (September 2010): 516–27.

2   Jason P. Block et al., "Consumers' Estimation of Calorie Content at Fast Food Restaurants: Cross Sectional Observational Study," *BMJ* (2013): 346:f2907.

3   eatright.org/Public/content.aspx?id=10936.

4   Brian Wansink and Pierre Chandon, "Can 'Low-Fat' Nutrition Labels Lead to Obesity?" *Journal of Marketing Research* 43, no. 4 (November 2006): 605–17.

5   fda.gov/NewsEvents/Newsroom/PressAnnouncements/ucm373939.htm.

Chapter 13: Vitamins and Supplements

1   "Position of the American Dietetic Association, Dietitians of Canada, and the American College of Sports Medicine: Nutrition and Athletic Performance," *Journal of the American Dietetic Association* 109 (2009): 509–27.

2   J. J. Otten et al., Institute of Medicine, "The Dietary Reference Intakes: The Essential Guide to Nutrient Requirements," Washington, DC: National Academies Press; 2006.

3   Kevin C. Maki et al., "Green Tea Catechin Consumption Enhances Exercise-Induced Abdominal Fat Loss in Overweight and Obese Adults," *Journal of Nutrition* 139, no. 2 (February 2009): 264–70.

Chapter 14: Adapting Mainstream Dieting Strategies to Run to Lose

1 L. A. Bazzano et al., "Effects of Low-Carbohydrate and Low-Fat Diets: A Randomized Trial," *Annals of Internal Medicine* 161 (2014): 309–18.

2 D. A. Weigle et al., "A High-Protein Diet Induces Sustained Reductions in Appetite, Ad Libitum Caloric Intake, and Body Weight Despite Compensatory Changes in Diurnal Plasma Leptin and Ghrelin Concentrations," *American Journal of Clinical Nutrition* 82, no.1 (July 2005): 41–48.

3 M. S. Westerterp-Plantenga et al., "High Protein Intake Sustains Weight Maintenance after Body Weight Loss in Humans," *International Journal of Obesity* 28 (2004): 57–64.

4 Johnstone et al., "Effects of High-Protein Ketogenic Diet on Hunger, Appetite, and Weight Loss in Obese Men Feeding Ad Libitum," *American Journal of Clinical Nutrition* 87, no. 1 (January 2008): 44–55.

5 S. M. Pasiakos et al., "Effects of High-Protein Diets on Fat-Free Mass and Muscle Protein Synthesis Following Weight Loss: A Randomized Clinical Trial," *FASEB Journal* 27, no. 9 (2013): 3837.

6 J. E. Flood-Obbagy and B. J. Rolls, "The Effect of Fruit in Different Forms on Energy Intake and Satiety at a Meal," *Appetite* 52, no. 2 (April 2009): 416–22. doi: 10.1016/j.appet.2008.12.001. Epub December 6, 2008.

7 N. Halberg et al., "Effect of Intermittent Fasting and Refeeding on Insulin Action in Healthy Men," *Journal of Applied Physiology* 99 (2005): 2128–36.

Chapter 15: Metabolism Basics

1 womenshealthmag.com/weight-loss/lazy-girl-weight-loss.

2 R. Ferraro et al., "Lower Sedentary Metabolic Rate in Women Compared with Men," *Journal of Clinical Investigation* 90, no. 3 (September 1992): 780–84.

3 Susan B. Roberts and Gerard E. Dallal, "Energy Requirements and Aging," *Public Health Nutrition* 8, no. 7A: 1028–36.

4 S. B. Roberts and I. Rosenberg, "Nutrition and Aging: Changes in the Regulation of Energy Metabolism with Aging," *Physiological Reviews* 86, no. 2 (April 2006): 651–67.

5 S. R. Davis et al., "Understanding Weight Gain at Menopause," *Climacteric: The Journal of the International Menopause Society* 15, no. 5: (2012): 419–29.

6 S. Santosa and M. D. Jensen, "Adipocyte Fatty Acid Storage Factors Enhance Subcutaneous Fat Storage in Postmenopausal Women," *Diabetes* 62, no. 3 (2012): 775.

7   B. Sternfeld and S. Dugan, "Physical Activity and Health during the Menopausal Transition," *Obstetrics and Gynecology Clinics of North America* 38, no. 3 (2011): 537–66.

8   Sanjay R. Patel et al., "Association between Reduced Sleep and Weight Gain in Women," *American Journal of Epidemiology* 164, no. 10 (November 15, 2006): 947–54.

9   K. Spiegel et al., "Brief Communication: Sleep Curtailment in Healthy Young Men Is Associated with Decreased Leptin Levels, Elevated Ghrelin Levels, and Increased Hunger and Appetite," *Annals of Internal Medicine* 141, no. 11: 846–50.

10 Rachel R. Markwald et al., "Impact of Insufficient Sleep on Total Daily Energy Expenditure, Food Intake, and Weight Gain," *Proceedings of the National Academy of Sciences* 110, no. 14: 5695 700.

11 R. Hursel et al., "The Effects of Catechin Rich Teas and Caffeine on Energy Expenditure and Fat Oxidation: A Meta-Analysis," *Obesity Reviews* 12, no. 7 (July 2011): e573-81. doi: 10.1111/j.1467-789X.2011.00862.x. Epub March 2, 2011.

12 M. Yoshioka et al., "Effects of Red Pepper Added to High-Fat and High-Carbohydrate Meals on Energy Metabolism and Substrate Utilization in Japanese Women," *British Journal of Nutrition* 80 (1998): 503–10; M. Yoshioka et al., "Effects of Red Pepper Diet on the Energy Metabolism in Men," *Journal of Nutrition Science and Vitaminology* 41 (1995), 647–56.

Chapter 16: Calculating How Many Calories You Need

1   A. M. Roza and H. M. Shizgal, "The Harris-Benedict Equation Reevaluated," *American Journal of Clinical Nutrition* 40, no. 1 (July 1984): 168–82.

2   M. D. Mifflin et al., "A New Predictive Equation for Resting Energy Expenditure in Healthy Individuals," *Journal of the American Dietetic Association* 51 (2005): 241–47.

3   ajcn.nutrition.org/content/79/5/921S.full.

Chapter 18: Avoiding GI Distress

1   Erick Prado de Oliveira, Roberto Carlos Burini, and Asker Jeukendrup, "Gastrointestinal Complaints during Exercise: Prevalence, Etiology, and Nutritional Recommendations," *Sports Medicine* 44, Suppl 1 (2014): S79–S85.

2   Ibid.

Chapter 20: Carb-Loading for Half-Marathons and Marathons

1 G. I. Atkinson et al., "Pre-Race Dietary Carbohydrate Intake Can Independently Influence Sub-Elite Marathon Running Performance," *International Journal of Sports Medicine* 32, no. 8 (August 2011): 611–17. Epub May 17, 2011.

Chapter 22: Eating for Recovery

1 D. R. Crabtree et al., "The Effects of High-Intensity Exercise on Neural Responses to Images of Food," *American Journal of Clinical Nutrition* 99, no. 2 (February 2014): 258–67.

Chapter 24: How to Burn More Calories While You Work Out

1 K. J. Sevits et al., "Total Daily Energy Expenditure Is Increased Following a Single Bout of Sprint Interval Training," *Physiology Reports* 1, no. 5 (October 2013): e00131.

2 A. M. Knab et al., "The Magnitude and Duration of Increased Energy Expenditure Following a 45-Minute Bout of Vigorous Exercise May Have Implications for Weight Loss and Management," *Medicine and Science in Sports and Exercise* 43, no. 9 (September 2011): 1643–48.

3 J. D. Bartlett, "High-Intensity Interval Running Is Perceived to Be More Enjoyable Than Moderate-Intensity Continuous Exercise: Implications for Exercise Adherence," *Journal of Sports Sciences* 29, no. 6 (March 2011): 547–53.

Chapter 25: Strength Training for Weight Loss

1 R. A. Mekary et al., "Weight Training, Aerobic Physical Activities, and Long-Term Waist Circumference Change in Men," *Obesity* 23 (2015): 461–67.

2 runnersworldonline.com.au/runners-strength-workout-can-done-anywhere/.

Chapter 28: Emotional Eating

1 S. H. Ahmed, K. Guillem, and Y. Vandaele, "Sugar Addiction: Pushing the Drug-Sugar Analogy to the Limit," *Current Opinion in Clinical Nutrition and Metabolic Care* 16, no. 4 (July 2013): 434–39.

2   Suzanne Higgs and Jessica Donahoe, "Focusing on Food during Lunch Enhances Lunch Memory and Decreases Later Snack Intake," *Appetite* 57, no. 1 (August 2011): 202–6.

3   Carolina O. C. Werle, Brian Wansink, and Collin R. Payne, "Is It Fun or Exercise? The Framing of Physical Activity Biases Subsequent Snacking," *Marketing Letters* (May 2014): http://link.springer.com/article/10.1007%2Fs11002-014-9301-6#page-1.

Chapter 29: How Stress Impacts Your Weight and Your Running Life

1   K. E. Rehm et al., "The Impact of Self-Reported Psychological Stress Levels on Changes to Peripheral Blood Immune Biomarkers in Recreational Marathon Runners during Training and Recovery," *Neuroimmunomodulation* 20, no. 3 (2013): 164–76.

2   Kirstin Aschbacher et al., "Chronic Stress Increases Vulnerability to Diet-Related Abdominal Fat, Oxidative Stress, and Metabolic Risk," *Psychoneuroendocrinology* 46 (August 2014): 14–22.

3   ucsf.edu/news/2014/04/113881/chronic-stress-heightens-vulnerability-diet-related-metabolic-risk.

4   R. Leproult et al., "Sleep Loss Results in an Elevation of Cortisol Levels the Next Evening," *Sleep* 20, no. 10 (October 1997): 865–70.

5   Jennifer Daubenmier et al., "Mindfulness Intervention for Stress Eating to Reduce Cortisol and Abdominal Fat among Overweight and Obese Women: An Exploratory Randomized Controlled Study," *Journal of Obesity* 2011 (2011): Article ID 651936.

Chapter 30: From Mindful to Mindless: How to Create Healthy Habits That Last for Life

1   David T. Neal, Wendy Wood, and Aimee Drolet, "How Do People Adhere to Goals When Willpower Is Low? The Profits (and Pitfalls) of Strong Habits," *Journal of Personality and Social Psychology* 104, no. 6 (June 2013): 959–75.

2   Gretchen Rubin, *Better Than Before: Mastering the Habits of Our Everyday Lives* (New York: Crown Publishers, 2015).

Food Label Quick-Reference Guide

1 Bidisha Mandal, "Use of Food Labels as a Weight-Loss Behavior," *Journal of Consumer Affairs* 44, no. 3 (September 2010): 516–27.

2 eatright.org/resource/food/nutrition/nutrition-facts-and-food-labels /the-basics-of-the-nutrition-facts-panel.

3 "Guidance for Industry: A Food Labeling Guide" (9.AppendixA: Definitions of Nutrient Content Claims) www.fda.gov/Food/GuidanceRegulation /GuidanceDocumentsRegulatoryInformation/LabelingNutrition /ucm2006828.htm.

INDEX

Boldface page references indicate illustrations.
Underscored references indicate tables or boxed text.

ABOUT THE AUTHORS

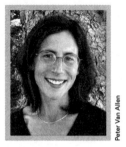

Peter Van Allen

Jennifer Van Allen is a freelance writer and running coach certified by USATF and RRCA. The former special projects editor for *Runner's World*, Van Allen has finished 49 marathons and ultramarathons. She lives in Portland, Maine.

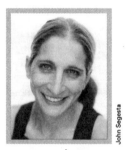

John Segesta

Pamela Nisevich Bede, RD, CSSD, is a sports nutrition expert and co-owner of Swim, Bike, Run, Eat!, LLC, a nutrition consulting firm.